Clinician's Guide to the Diagnosis and Management of Tooth Sensitivity

Sahar Taha • Brian H. Clarkson
Editors

Clinician's Guide to the Diagnosis and Management of Tooth Sensitivity

Springer

Editors
Sahar Taha
Department of Conservative Dentistry
Faculty of Dentistry
University of Jordan
Amman
Jordan

Brian H. Clarkson
Department of Cariology, Restorative
Sciences and Endodontics
University of Michigan School
of Dentistry
Ann Arbor, MI
USA

ISBN 978-3-642-45163-8 ISBN 978-3-642-45164-5 (eBook)
DOI 10.1007/978-3-642-45164-5
Springer Heidelberg New York Dordrecht London

Library of Congress Control Number: 2014932539

Printed on acid-free paper

Springer is part of Springer Science+Business Media (www.springer.com)

Contents

1 Introduction to Dentin Hypersensitivity

Sahar Taha

Abstract

Dentin hypersensitivity was defined as "a short, sharp pain arising from exposed dentin in response to stimuli typically thermal, evaporative, tactile, osmotic or chemical and which cannot be ascribed to any other form of dental defect or disease." In this chapter, characteristics of this condition are discussed in addition to its prevalence reported using different methods of diagnosis. The epidemiology of the condition, its impact on the patient's oral health quality of life, and how to measure it are also discussed.

1.1 Definition

The Canadian advisory board on dentin hypersensitivity (2003) defined it as "a short, sharp pain arising from exposed dentin in response to stimuli typically thermal, evaporative, tactile, osmotic or chemical and which cannot be ascribed to any other form of dental defect or disease."

A similar definition was suggested by Pashley (1994): "a sharp, transient, well-localized pain in response to tactile, thermal, evaporative, or osmotic stimuli, which does not occur spontaneously and does not persist after removal of the stimuli."

Carefully analyzing the definition, one can deduce the following characteristics of this condition:

- Sharp transient pain.
- Stimulated pain (thermal, evaporative, tactile, osmotic, or chemical).
- Occurs when dentin is exposed.
- Diagnosis includes the exclusion of other dental defects or diseases.

Dentin hypersensitivity has been described as the "common cold of dentistry" by some and "toothbrush disease" by others, when it occurs in the presence of gingival recession (Pashley et al. 2008).

1.2 Prevalence of DH

Contrary to what is generally believed, the literature on the prevalence of DH is not abundant (Splieth and Tachou 2012), although DH seems to be a common condition among adult population

S. Taha, DDS, MS, Diplomate (ABOD)
Department of Conservative Dentistry,
Faculty of Dentistry, University of Jordan,
13795, Amman 11942, Jordan
e-mail: shr_taha@yahoo.com, staha@ju.edu.jo

S. Taha, B.H. Clarkson (eds.), *Clinician's Guide to the Diagnosis and Management of Tooth Sensitivity*,
DOI 10.1007/978-3-642-45164-5_1, © Springer-Verlag Berlin Heidelberg 2014

with prevalence values ranging from 1.34 to 98 % (Table 1.1). The diversity in the reported prevalence values is primarily attributed to the difference in sample selection and in the methods used to diagnose DH (Splieth and Tachou 2012; Lin and Gillam 2012; Dababneh et al. 1999). Questionnaires and clinical examination are the methods most commonly used. Studies that relied on questionnaires only to diagnose DH yielded higher values of prevalence than those combined with clinical examination (Table 1.1). In 2004, Rees and Addy carried out a cross-sectional study of buccal cervical sensitivity in a UK general practice population and reviewed studies on DH prevalence. They suggested reasons for the variability of prevalence values reported in the literature, including the different study designs used to assess the condition; variation in patients' oral hygiene habits; consumption of erosive foods and drinks; and the type of setting where the study was carried out. Questionnaires used in different studies involved questions evaluating three aspects of DH: questions related to pain or discomfort experienced by the patient, oral hygiene habits, periodontal treatment, and discomfort following this treatment. A question to evaluate possible erosive factors was also added by some investigators (Gillam et al. 2001; Clayton et al. 2002). The use of questionnaires that require self-reporting of DH may well overestimate the magnitude of the problem, because of sensitivity caused by other pathologies, such as caries and cracked tooth syndrome (Rees and Addy 2004). Studies carried out at hospitals or specialty practices tend to report higher prevalence values, presumably because of the greater risk of root exposure as a result of periodontal attachment loss and gingival recession following periodontal treatment.

Taking all this into consideration, it seems prudent to divide the prevalence of this condition into three categories: *DH prevalence using surveys (around 50 %); DH prevalence diagnosed using combined surveys and clinical exams (15–20 %); and DH in patients who have periodontal disease or have been receiving periodontal treatment (60–90 %)*. Referring back to the definition of DH previously mentioned, the latest category might reflect a different etiology and should not be considered when reporting prevalence of the condition. Bacteria were reported to penetrate dentin to a considerable distance in periodontally diseased teeth (Adriaens et al. 1988). Such sensitivity of dentin therefore is a separate clinical entity possibly requiring different preventive and management strategies (Dababneh et al. 1999).

There was a significant association between DH and patients who received periodontal treatment, surgical and nonsurgical (Fischer et al. 1992), and in patients who had gingival recession (Tammaro et al. 2000; Taani and Awartani 2001; Chabanski et al. 1997; Rees et al. 2003). Furthermore, higher prevalence values were reported among patients referred to periodontology clinics than the general practice clinics (Chabanski et al. 1997). This would suggest a significant role of periodontal disease in the etiology of DH (Rees et al. 2003).

Many studies associated an increased prevalence of DH with gingival recession (Al-Wahadni and Linden 2002; Dhaliwal et al. 2012). A much higher proportion (65 %) of the DH group had gingival recession of ≥3 mm compared with only 34 % of the control group ($P < 0.0001$).

The incidence of DH increases after periodontal treatment (Splieth and Tachou 2012). Al-Sabbagh et al. found that the incidence increased from 30 % preoperatively to 79 % after 1 week of open-flap periodontal debridement (Al-Sabbagh et al. 2010). Furthermore, Fischer et al. (1991) found that supragingival and subgingival scaling might cause a transient occurrence of DH. In a systematic review carried out by Lin and Gillam (2012), the reported prevalence for DH following nonsurgical therapy was between 62.5 and 90 % 1 day after treatment decreasing to approximately 52.6–55 % after 1 week. The prevalence of DH following surgical therapy was between 76.8 and 80.4 % 1 day after treatment subsequently decreasing over time to 36.8 % after 1 week, 33.4 % after 2 weeks, 29.6 % after 4 weeks, and 21.7 % after 8 weeks. It was suggested that DH may be relatively mild/moderate in nature and transient in duration after periodontal therapy.

Table 1.1 Summary of prevalence studies on DH among attendees of general dental practices or hospitals

Study	Country	*n*	Study type	Method of clinical assessment	Setting	Prevalence (%)	Peak of age	M:F ratio	Commonly affected teeth	% with GR[a]
Clayton et al. (2002)	UK	250	Q[b]	NA[i]	GDP[f]	50	3rd decade	1:1	Mand[h] right sextant	NA
Gillam et al. (2001)	UK and Korea	557	Q	NA	GDP	52–55.4	3rd–4th decades	NA	NA	NA
Gillam et al. (1999)	UK	277	Q	NA	GDP	52	3rd decade	1:1.4	NA	NA
Bamise et al. (2007)	Nigeria	2,165	Q+CE[c]	AB[d]/Probing	University	1.34	4th decade	1.4:1	Molars	12.8 %
Rees and Addy (2004)	UK	5,477	Q+CE	AB/PDA[e]	GDP	2.8	4th decade	1:1.5	Max[g] 1st molars	93 %
Taani and Awartani (2001)	Saudi Arabia	259	Q+CE	AB/PDA	GDP	GDP 42.4	4th decade	GDP 1:4	Max molars and mand anteriors	5 %
Fischer et al. (1992)	Brazil	635	Q+CE	AB/Probing	Marine dental clinic	17	M: 6th, F: 3rd decade	1:1	Incisors and premolars	NA
Flynn et al. (1985)	Scotland	369	Q+CE	CWMR[j]/Probing	University	8.7	4th decade	1:1	Premolars	NA
Liu et al. (1998)	Taiwan	780	Q+CE	AB/Probing	University	32	NA	1:1	Premolars and molars	23 %
Amarasena et al. (2011)	Australia	12,692	Q+CE	NA	GDP	9.1	4th–5th decades	1:1.5	Max premolars and molars	39 %
Chrysanthakopoulos (2011)	Greece	1,450	Q+CE	AB	GDP	18.2	5th in males 7th in females	1:1.25	Premolars	85.9 %
Ye et al. (2012)	China	2,120	Q+CE	AB	GDP	34.1	5th decade	1:1.5	Premolars	84.3 %
Tengrungsun et al. (2012)	Thailand	420	Q+CE	AB	University	30.7	4th decade	1:2.4	1st molar	NA
Bahsi et al. (2012)	Turkey	1,368	Q+CE	AB/Probing	GDP	5.3	5th decade	1:2	Max premolars	88.4 %
Dhaliwal et al. (2012)	Punjab, India	650	Q+CE	AB	Screening participants in villages	25	6th decade	1:1.6	Mand incisors	NA
Cunha-Cruz et al. (2013)	USA	787	Q+CE	AB	GDP	12.3	18–44	1:2.6	Premolars and molars	85.6 %

[a]Gingival recession
[b]Questionnaire
[c]Clinical examination
[d]Sensitivity to air blast
[e]Periodontal disease assessment
[f]General dental practice
[g]Maxillary
[h]Mandibular
[i]Not applicable
[j]Cold water mouth rinse

1.3 Distribution

The condition is mostly prevalent among the young population in the 3rd and 4th decades (Table 1.1). The prevalence may shift in the future to a younger age group because of the increase in acidic food/drink intake and the influence of greater oral hygiene awareness and measures (Chabanski et al. 1997; Clayton et al. 2002).

In general, a slightly higher prevalence of DH was reported in females than in males, which may reflect their better oral hygiene awareness (Dababneh et al. 1999). This difference was not statistically significant in the majority of the studies.

Various intraoral locations can be affected with DH. Sites of predilection in descending order are canines and first premolars, incisors and second premolars, and molars (Dababneh et al. 1999). However, the literature has not been consistent in reporting the intraoral distribution of the condition (Bamise et al. 2007). The buccal surface seems to be the most affected, followed by labial, occlusal, distal, and lingual. Incisal and palatal surfaces were the least affected (Splieth and Tachou 2012; Amarasena et al. 2011).

1.4 Dentin Hypersensitivity Impact on Quality of Life

Prevalence values reported in all the previously mentioned studies relied on clinical tests or questionnaires to assess the symptoms associated with DH. However, the quality of life of DH patients has been widely underestimated or unrecognized. The depth and complexity of pain experiences associated with sensitivity impacts on functional status and everyday activities such as eating, drinking, talking, tooth brushing, and social interaction. It also has a subtle impact on emotions and identity (Boiko et al. 2010). Dentin hypersensitivity interfered with eating 31 % of the time, 41.4 % with brushing, and 72.4 % with drinking water (Bamise et al. 2007).

Quality of life research has gained more popularity and attention in recent years in the medical field. It is now at the forefront of public health policies (Bekes and Hirsch 2012). Quality of life can be defined as "an individual's perception of his/her position in life, in the context of the culture and value systems in which he/she lives and in relation to his/her expectations, goals and concerns" (Study protocol for the World Health Organization project to develop a Quality of Life assessment instrument (WHOQOL) 1993).

Oral health-related quality of life (OHRQoL) is a part of the health-related quality of life that focuses on oral health and orofacial concerns. It describes the way in which oral health affects a person's ability to function, psychological status, social factors, and pain or discomfort (Bekes and Hirsch 2012). Although pain evaluation with clinical tests has been widely employed in clinical practice, subjective pain evaluation through OHRQoL may influence whether and how patients should be treated (Bekes et al. 2009). Dentin hypersensitivity can have a negative impact on the patients' OHRQoL (Bekes and Hirsch 2012).

Over the years, the oral health impact profile (OHIP) tool has been widely used to evaluate the impact of dental conditions on the patient's well-being. However, many OHIP items are irrelevant to specific oral health states (Wong et al. 2007). A condition-specific Dentin Hypersensitivity Experience Questionnaire (DHEQ) was developed by Boiko et al. (2010), which was based on a multistaged impact approach and proper validation. This 48-item questionnaire showed good psychometric properties in both a general population and a clinical sample, enabling better understanding of the subjective nature of the condition. A short form of this questionnaire was also tested (Annex 1.1).

1.5 Annex 1.1 Dental Sensitivity Experience Questionnaire 15 Items (DHEQ-15)*

Thinking about yourself over the last month to what extent would you agree or disagree with the following statements: (Please tick only one response for each question)

1. Having sensations in my teeth takes a lot of the pleasure out of eating and drinking.
   - ☐ Strongly agree (7)
   - ☐ Agree (6)
   - ☐ Agree a Little (5)
   - ☐ Neither agree or disagree (4)
   - ☐ Disagree a little (3)
   - ☐ Disagree (2)
   - ☐ Strongly disagree (1)

2. It takes a long time to finish some foods and drinks because of sensations in my teeth.
   - ☐ Strongly agree (7)
   - ☐ Agree (6)
   - ☐ Agree a little (5)
   - ☐ Neither agree or disagree (4)
   - ☐ Disagree a little (3)
   - ☐ Disagree (2)
   - ☐ Strongly disagree (1)

3. There have been times when I have had problems eating ice cream because of these sensations.
   - ☐ Strongly agree (7)
   - ☐ Agree (6)
   - ☐ Agree a little (5)
   - ☐ Neither agree or disagree (4)
   - ☐ Disagree a little (3)
   - ☐ Disagree (2)
   - ☐ Strongly disagree (1)

4. I have to change the way I eat or drink certain things
   - ☐ Strongly agree (7)
   - ☐ Agree (6)
   - ☐ Agree a little (5)
   - ☐ Neither agree or disagree (4)
   - ☐ Disagree a little (3)
   - ☐ Disagree (2)
   - ☐ Strongly disagree (1)

5. I have to be careful how I breathe on a cold day.
   - ☐ Strongly agree (7)
   - ☐ Agree (6)
   - ☐ Agree a little (5)
   - ☐ Neither agree or disagree (4)
   - ☐ Disagree a little (3)
   - ☐ Disagree (2)
   - ☐ Strongly disagree (1)

6. When eating some foods I have made sure they don't touch certain teeth.
   - ☐ Strongly agree (7)
   - ☐ Agree (6)
   - ☐ Agree a little (5)
   - ☐ Neither agree or disagree (4)
   - ☐ Disagree a little (3)
   - ☐ Disagree (2)
   - ☐ Strongly disagree (1)

*Machuca C, Baker SR, Robinson PG (2013) Development and validation of the short-form of the Dentine Hypersensitivity Experience Questionnaire (DHEQ). Presented at International Association for Dental Research, Seattle, 2013

7. Because of the sensations I take longer than others to finish a meal.
   - ☐ Strongly agree (7)
   - ☐ Agree (6)
   - ☐ Agree a little (5)
   - ☐ Neither agree or disagree (4)
   - ☐ Disagree a little (3)
   - ☐ Disagree (2)
   - ☐ Strongly disagree (1)

8. I have to be careful what I eat when I am with others because of the sensations in my teeth.
   - ☐ Strongly agree (7)
   - ☐ Agree (6)
   - ☐ Agree a little (5)
   - ☐ Neither agree or disagree (4)
   - ☐ Disagree a little (3)
   - ☐ Disagree (2)
   - ☐ Strongly disagree (1)

9. Going to the dentist is hard for me because I know it is going to be painful as a result of sensations in my teeth.
   - ☐ Strongly agree (7)
   - ☐ Agree (6)
   - ☐ Agree a little (5)
   - ☐ Neither agree or disagree (4)
   - ☐ Disagree a little (3)
   - ☐ Disagree (2)
   - ☐ Strongly disagree (1)

10. I've been anxious that something I eat or drink might cause sensations in my teeth.
   - ☐ Strongly agree (7)
   - ☐ Agree (6)
   - ☐ Agree a little (5)
   - ☐ Neither agree or disagree (4)
   - ☐ Disagree a little (3)
   - ☐ Disagree (2)
   - ☐ Strongly disagree (1)

11. The sensations in my teeth have been irritating.
   - ☐ Strongly agree (7)
   - ☐ Agree (6)
   - ☐ Agree a little (5)
   - ☐ Neither agree or disagree (4)
   - ☐ Disagree a little (3)
   - ☐ Disagree (2)
   - ☐ Strongly disagree (1)

12. The sensations in my teeth have been annoying.
   - ☐ Strongly agree (7)
   - ☐ Agree (6)
   - ☐ Agree a little (5)
   - ☐ Neither agree or disagree (4)
   - ☐ Disagree a little (3)
   - ☐ Disagree (2)
   - ☐ Strongly disagree (1)

13. Having these sensations in my teeth makes me feel old.
   - ☐ Strongly agree (7)
   - ☐ Agree (6)
   - ☐ Agree a little (5)
   - ☐ Neither agree or disagree (4)
   - ☐ Disagree a little (3)
   - ☐ Disagree (2)
   - ☐ Strongly disagree (1)

14. Having these sensations in my teeth makes me feel damaged.
   - ☐ Strongly agree (7)
   - ☐ Agree (6)
   - ☐ Agree a little (5)
   - ☐ Neither agree or disagree (4)
   - ☐ Disagree a little (3)
   - ☐ Disagree (2)
   - ☐ Strongly disagree (1)

15. Having these sensations in my teeth makes me feel though I am unhealthy.
   - ☐ Strongly agree (7)
   - ☐ Agree (6)
   - ☐ Agree a little (5)
   - ☐ Neither agree or disagree (4)
   - ☐ Disagree a little (3)
   - ☐ Disagree (2)
   - ☐ Strongly disagree (1)

References

Adriaens PA, Edwards CA, De Boever JA, Loesche WJ (1988) Ultrastructural observations on bacterial invasion in cementum and radicular dentin of periodontally diseased human teeth. J Periodontol 59(8): 493–503

Al-Sabbagh M, Beneduce C, Andreana S, Ciancio SG (2010) Incidence and time course of dentinal hypersensitivity after periodontal surgery. Gen Dent 58(1):e14–e19

Al-Wahadni A, Linden GJ (2002) Dentine hypersensitivity in Jordanian dental attenders. A case control study. J Clin Periodontol 29(8):688–693, cpe290804 [pii]

Amarasena N, Spencer J, Ou Y, Brennan D (2011) Dentine hypersensitivity in a private practice patient population in Australia. J Oral Rehabil 38(1):52–60. doi:10.1111/j.1365-2842.2010.02132.x, JOR2132 [pii]

Bahsi E, Dalli M, Uzgur R, Turkal M, Hamidi MM, Colak H (2012) An analysis of the aetiology, prevalence and clinical features of dentine hypersensitivity in a general dental population. Eur Rev Med Pharmacol Sci 16(8):1107–1116

Bamise CT, Olusile AO, Oginni AO, Dosumu OO (2007) The prevalence of dentine hypersensitivity among adult patients attending a Nigerian teaching hospital. Oral Health Prev Dent 5(1):49–53

Bekes K, Hirsch C (2012) What is known about the influence of dentine hypersensitivity on oral health-related quality of life? Clin Oral Investig. doi:10.1007/s00784-012-0888-9

Bekes K, John MT, Schaller HG, Hirsch C (2009) Oral health-related quality of life in patients seeking care for dentin hypersensitivity. J Oral Rehabil 36(1):45–51. doi:10.1111/j.1365-2842.2008.01901.x, JOR1901 [pii]

Boiko OV, Baker SR, Gibson BJ, Locker D, Sufi F, Barlow AP, Robinson PG (2010) Construction and validation of the quality of life measure for dentine hypersensitivity (DHEQ). J Clin Periodontol 37(11):973–980. doi:10.1111/j.1600-051X.2010.01618.x

Canadian Advisory Board on Dentin Hypersensitivity (2003) Consensus-based recommendations for the diagnosis and management of dentin hypersensitivity. J Can Dent Assoc 69(4):221–226

Chabanski MB, Gillam DG, Bulman JS, Newman HN (1997) Clinical evaluation of cervical dentine sensitivity in a population of patients referred to a specialist periodontology department: a pilot study. J Oral Rehabil 24(9):666–672

Chrysanthakopoulos NA (2011) Prevalence of dentine hypersensitivity in a general dental practice in Greece. J Clin Exp Dent 3(5):e445–e451

Clayton DR, McCarthy D, Gillam DG (2002) A study of the prevalence and distribution of dentine sensitivity in a population of 17-58-year-old serving personnel on an RAF base in the Midlands. J Oral Rehabil 29(1):14–23, 805 [pii]

Cunha-Cruz J, Wataha JC, Heaton LJ, Rothen M, Sobieraj M, Scott J, Berg J (2013) The prevalence of dentin hypersensitivity in general dental practices in the northwest United States. J Am Dent Assoc 144(3):288–296, 144/3/288 [pii]

Dababneh RH, Khouri AT, Addy M (1999) Dentine hypersensitivity – an enigma? A review of terminology, mechanisms, aetiology and management. Br Dent J 187(11):606–611; discussion 603. doi:10.1038/sj.bdj.4800345a, 4800345a [pii]

Dhaliwal JS, Palwankar P, Khinda PK, Sodhi SK (2012) Prevalence of dentine hypersensitivity: a cross-sectional study in rural Punjabi Indians. J Indian Soc Periodontol 16(3):426–429. doi:10.4103/0972-124X.100924, JISP-16-426 [pii]

Fischer C, Wennberg A, Fischer RG, Attstrom R (1991) Clinical-evaluation of pulp and dentin sensitivity after supragingival and subgingival scaling. Endod Dent Traumatol 7(6):259–265

Fischer C, Fischer RG, Wennberg A (1992) Prevalence and distribution of cervical dentine hypersensitivity in a population in Rio de Janeiro. Brazil J Dent 20(5):272–276, 0300-5712(92)90043-C [pii]

Flynn J, Galloway R, Orchardson R (1985) The incidence of 'hypersensitive' teeth in the West of Scotland. J Dent 13(3):230–236

Gillam DG, Seo HS, Bulman JS, Newman HN (1999) Perceptions of dentine hypersensitivity in a general practice population. J Oral Rehabil 26(9):710–714, jor436 [pii]

Gillam DG, Seo HS, Newman HN, Bulman JS (2001) Comparison of dentine hypersensitivity in selected occidental and oriental populations. J Oral Rehabil 28(1):20–25, jor631 [pii]

Lin YH, Gillam DG (2012) The prevalence of root sensitivity following periodontal therapy: a systematic review. Int J Dent 2012:407023. doi:10.1155/2012/407023

Liu HC, Lan WH, Hsieh CC (1998) Prevalence and distribution of cervical dentin hypersensitivity in a population in Taipei, Taiwan. J Endod 24(1):45–47. doi:10.1016/S0099-2399(98)80213-6, S0099-2399(98)80213-6 [pii]

Pashley DH (1994) Theory of dentin sensitivity. J Clin Dent 5 Spec No:65–67

Pashley DH, Tay FR, Haywood VB, Collins MA, Drisko CL (2008) Consensus-based recommendations for the diagnosis and management of dentin hypersensitivity. Inside Dentistry 4(9 (Special Issue)):1–35

Rees JS, Addy M (2004) A cross-sectional study of buccal cervical sensitivity in UK general dental practice and a summary review of prevalence studies. Int J Dent Hyg 2(2):64–69. doi:10.1111/j.1601-5029.2004.00068.x, IDH068 [pii]

Rees JS, Jin LJ, Lam S, Kudanowska I, Vowles R (2003) The prevalence of dentine hypersensitivity in a hospital clinic population in Hong Kong. J Dent 31(7):453–461, S0300571203000927 [pii]

Splieth CH, Tachou A (2012) Epidemiology of dentin hypersensitivity. Clin Oral Investig. doi:10.1007/s00784-012-0889-8

Study protocol for the World Health Organization project to develop a Quality of Life assessment instrument (WHOQOL) (1993) Qual Life Res 2(2):153–159

Taani DQ, Awartani F (2001) Prevalence and distribution of dentin hypersensitivity and plaque in a dental hospital population. Quintessence Int 32(5):372–376

Tammaro S, Wennstrom JL, Bergenholtz G (2000) Root-dentin sensitivity following non-surgical periodontal treatment. J Clin Periodontol 27(9):690–697. doi:10.1034/j.1600-051x.2000.027009690.x

Tengrungsun T, Jamornnium Y, Tengrungsun S (2012) Prevalence of dentine hypersensitivity among Thai dental patients at the Faculty of Dentistry, Mahidol University. Southeast Asian J Trop Med Public Health 43(4):1059–1064

Wong AH, Cheung CS, McGrath C (2007) Developing a short form of Oral Health Impact Profile (OHIP) for dental aesthetics: OHIP-aesthetic. Community Dent Oral Epidemiol 35(1):64–72. doi:10.1111/j.1600-0528.2007.00330.x, COM330 [pii]

Ye W, Feng XP, Li R (2012) The prevalence of dentine hypersensitivity in Chinese adults. J Oral Rehabil 39(3):-182–187. doi:10.1111/j.1365-2842.2011.02248.x

2 "How Can Sensitive Dentin Become Hypersensitive?"

David H. Pashley

Abstract

When dentinal tubules first become exposed, patients note that those areas become more sensitive to tactile, evaporative, and osmotic stimuli. However, over time, especially with poor plaque control, those areas become progressively truly hypersensitive. There are a number of mechanisms responsible for hypersensitivity including localized pulpal inflammation, sprouting of pulpal nerves, and expression of "inflammatory" sodium channels. Often such hypersensitivity spontaneously disappears. These protective mechanisms will be reviewed. The problem arises for patients whose exposed dentin becomes hypersensitive and whose endogenous protective mechanism fails to correct the hypersensitivity.

2.1 Introduction

Brännström's (1962, 1992) hydrodynamic theory of dentin sensitivity proposed that hydrodynamic stimuli (hot or cold, tactile, evaporative or osmotic) caused sudden minute shifts of dentinal fluid that activate pulpal mechanoreceptors (Fig. 2.1) to cause sharp, well-localized tooth pain, thought to be due to A-delta sensory nerves (Narhi et al., 1992). A corollary of the hydrodynamic theory of pain is that anything that reduces dentin hydraulic conductance should decrease dentin sensitivity. Conversely, anything that increases dentin hydraulic conductance should increase dentin sensitivity. In this model, dentin hypersensitivity is equated with hyperconductance of dentinal fluid through tubules. In such a simple model, all things staying constant, increases in fluid flow should cause increases in dentin sensitivity. Unfortunately, all things do not stay constant.

2.2 Fluid Flow Models of Sensitivity

Our group was the first to report dentinal fluid flow across dog dentin in vivo (Pashley et al. 1981). In that same paper, we reported pulpal tissue pressures in dogs of 15–47 cm H_2O and that dentinal fluid flow was driven by pulpal tissue pressure (Fig. 2.2). This was later confirmed in humans in vivo (Ciucchi et al. 1995). In that paper, we reported pulpal tissue pressures of

D.H. Pashley, DMD, PhD
Department of Oral Biology,
College of Dental Medicine, Georgia Regents University,
1120 15th Street, CL-2112, Augusta, GA 30912, USA
e-mail: dpashley@gru.edu

S. Taha, B.H. Clarkson (eds.), *Clinician's Guide to the Diagnosis and Management of Tooth Sensitivity*,
DOI 10.1007/978-3-642-45164-5_2, © Springer-Verlag Berlin Heidelberg 2014

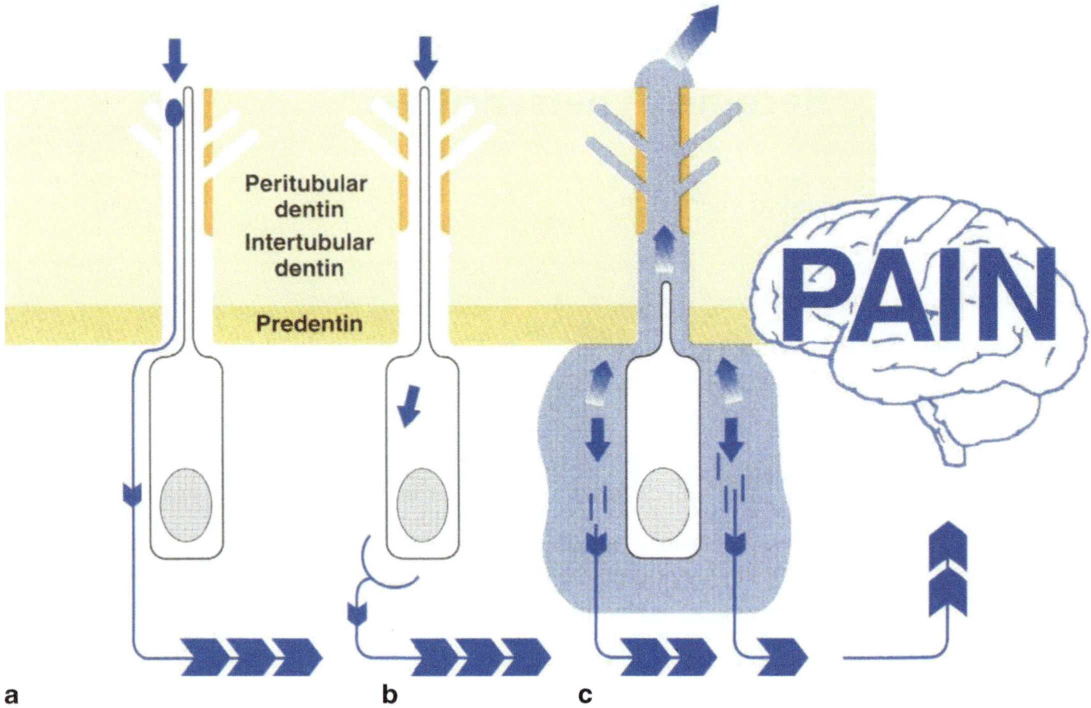

Fig. 2.1 Theories of dental pain. (**a**) Old theory that pulpal nerves extended out to the DEJ and made the DEJ sensitive. However, careful histology failed to demonstrate nerves at the DEJ. (**b**) In the 1950s, scientists thought that pulpal nerves synapsed with odontoblasts and that odontoblast processes extended to the DEJ. Careful histology revealed that odontoblast processes do not extend to the DEJ. (**c**) The hydrodynamic theory of dentin pain is that movements of dentinal fluid in tubules in either direction activate mechanoreceptor nerves in the pulp to cause dentin sensitivity (From Ten Cate (1998), p. 191 with permission)

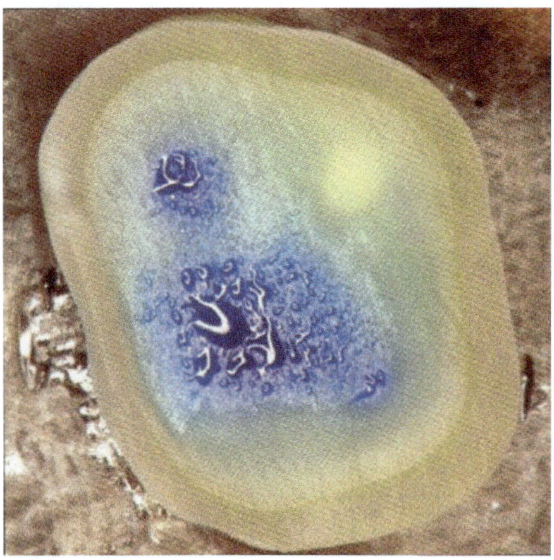

Fig. 2.2 Flattened occlusal surface of a tooth in vitro filled with blue dye that slowly seeps across open dentinal tubules under a pulpal tissue pressure of 20 cm H_2O. The tubules over pulp horns are shorter and are located closer together, making these tubules very sensitive (From Pashley and Tay (2012), with permission)

14–15 cm of water that was similar to pulpal tissue pressure in cats of 16 cm H_2O reported by Vongsavan and Matthews (1992). Vongsavan and Matthews actually calculated the velocity of outward movement of dentinal fluid in cat dentin at 1.4 μm s^{-1}. This outward seepage of dentinal fluid flow occurs because the pulpal tissue pressure is 16 cm H_2O greater than atmospheric pressure in normal pulps. This slow outward fluid flow is too slow to activate pulpal nerves. Using radioactive ^{125}I, Pashley and Matthews (1993) confirmed that outward directed convective fluid flow could significantly restrict the inward diffusion of small molecules. After Nissan et al. (1995) showed that bacterial endotoxin can diffuse through human dentin, Puapichartdumcong et al. (2005) reported that outwardly directed fluid flow under 15 cm H_2O pressure could significantly lower the flux of endotoxin across dentin. Thus, although outward fluid flow reduces inward diffusion, it does not eliminate it.

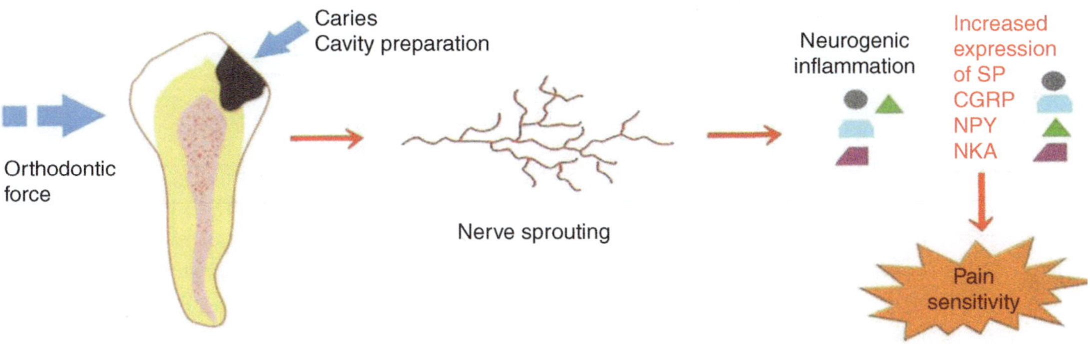

Fig. 2.3 Although this figure shows neuronal responses of the pulpodentin complex to caries, cavity preparation, or orthodontic tooth movement, many authorities believe that hypersensitive pulps undergo the same responses to inflammatory mediators (From Fouad (2012), with permission)

2.3 Effects of Inflammation of the Pulp

During pulpal inflammation, a large number of chemical mediators of inflammation are released, including histamine and serotonin, complement activation, and bradykinin release (Fouad 2012). Many of the mediators make pulpal nerves more sensitive than normal and cause the surrounding fibroblasts to divide more rapidly than normal. Fibroblasts release more nerve growth factor (NGF) that, in turn, causes nerve terminals to sprout and increase their neuropeptide content. This increase in nerve density is thought to be associated with the development of dentin hypersensitivity (Fig. 2.3). A receptive field in dentin is all of the dentinal tubules innervated by a single nerve and its branches. An increased size of receptive fields in inflamed pulps has been reported (Byers and Närhi 1999). Most of the nerves that sprout contain calcitonin gene-related product (CGRP) and substance P (SP). Both neuropeptides are known to vasodilate pulpal blood vessels and increase capillary permeability. These reactions lead to increases in tissue pressure (Heyeraas and Kvinnsland 1992; Berggren and Heyeraas 1999) and in outward fluid flow. This increase in outward fluid flow occurs not because dentin is more hyperconductive, but because of increases in local tissue pressure, the driving force for dentin fluid flow (Pashley 1992). As this fluid flows through narrow tissue spaces between pulpal nerves and dentin, the local shear forces on mechanoreceptors may bring the resting membrane potential of pulpal nerves closer to threshold, making them "hypersensitive" (Fig. 2.4). Working in cats in vivo, Matthews and Vongsavan (1994) reported that application of a negative pressure of −300 mmHg caused outward fluid flow to increase from 1.4 to 25 $\mu m\ s^{-1}$ to fire pulpal mechanoreceptors. They calculated that fluid flow rates >1.5 $nl\ s^{-1}\ mm^{-2}$ were required to activate intradental nerves in anesthetized cats.

2.4 Effects of Inflammation on Sodium Channels in Nerves

Inflammation also modifies the types of sodium channels that are distributed in sensory nerves. Sodium channels can be classified as tetrodotoxin sensitive or tetrodotoxin (TTX) resistant. When nerves are surrounded by inflammatory mediators, they not only sprout, they also upregulate new sodium channels (Na_v 1.8 and 1.9) that seem to be more easily activated (Fig. 2.5) than is seen in the absence of inflammation (Renton et al. 2005; Wells et al. 2007; Luo et al. 2008; Warren et al. 2008; Henry et al. 2009). Thus, in clinical cases of dentin hypersensitivity, if patients cannot successfully remove bacterial plaque on exposed hypersensitive dentin, that dentin may remain hypersensitive until some tubule occluding agent can reduce in inward flux of plaque products. These bacterial products sustain the localized pulpal inflammation, which

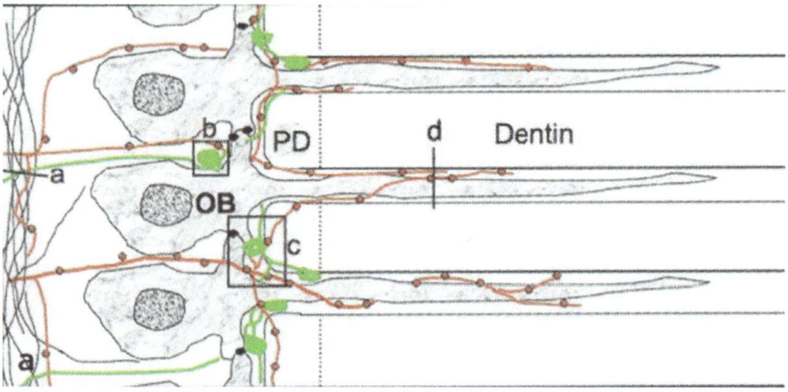

Fig. 2.4 Schematic of odontoblasts extending cellular processes out into deep dentin. Nerves in *red* (C-fibers) contain peptide neurotransmitters, substance P, and calcitonin gene-related peptide (CGRP). The larger *green* nerves are A-**δ** sensory nerves that carry sharp, well-localized pain of dentin sensitivity. *OB* designates the cell body of an odontoblast; *PD* designates the presence of predentin interposed between the odontoblast layer on the *left*, and mineralized dentin on the *right* (From Byers et al. (2012), p. 136)

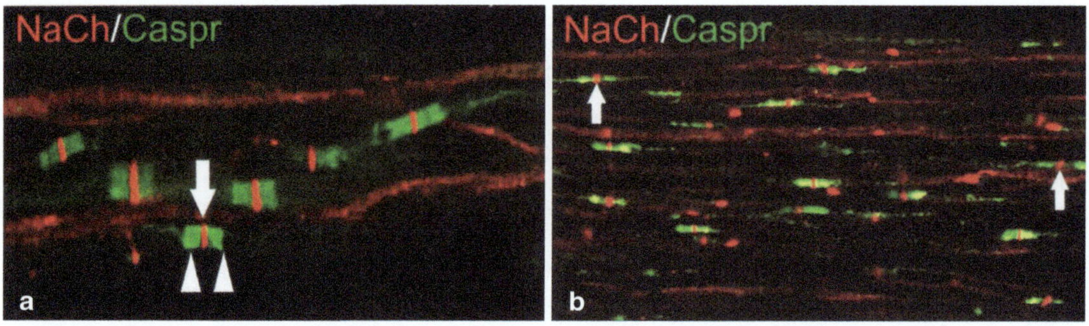

Fig. 2.5 (**a**) Confocal micrographs of sodium channels (*red*) Na_v 1.7 and Na_v 1.8 in pulpal axons and Caspr (*green*) that identify nodes of Ranvier in mylinated nerves in normal pulp. (**b**) On the *right* panel are shown those same neural proteins in inflammed pulps. Note the presence of more nerves in painful pulps (From Byers et al. (2012), p. 124)

makes pulpal nerves hypersensitive to hydrodynamic stimuli that might not normally cause pain.

Partial or complete tubule occlusion is an important part of treating dentin hypersensitivity, but plaque control is also very important. Tubule occluding agents may be more effective clinically if they include antibacterial agents that can control plaque.

When dentin is freshly exposed, it is very sensitive, even when the underlying pulp is healthy. However, if the freshly exposed dentin becomes covered with bacterial plaque, the tooth becomes hypersensitive when the pulps show signs of local inflammation beneath the exposed dentinal tubules (Lundy and Stanley 1969). What is in bacterial plaque that causes exposed dentin to become hypersensitive?

2.5 Effects of Bacterial Products on the Pulp

In 1962, Brännström recruited teenaged children whose premolars were scheduled for extraction for their orthodontic treatment. Under local anesthesia, he ground through the enamel of those premolars into the mid-coronal dentin to expose 5–10 mm^2 of dentin covered by smear layer

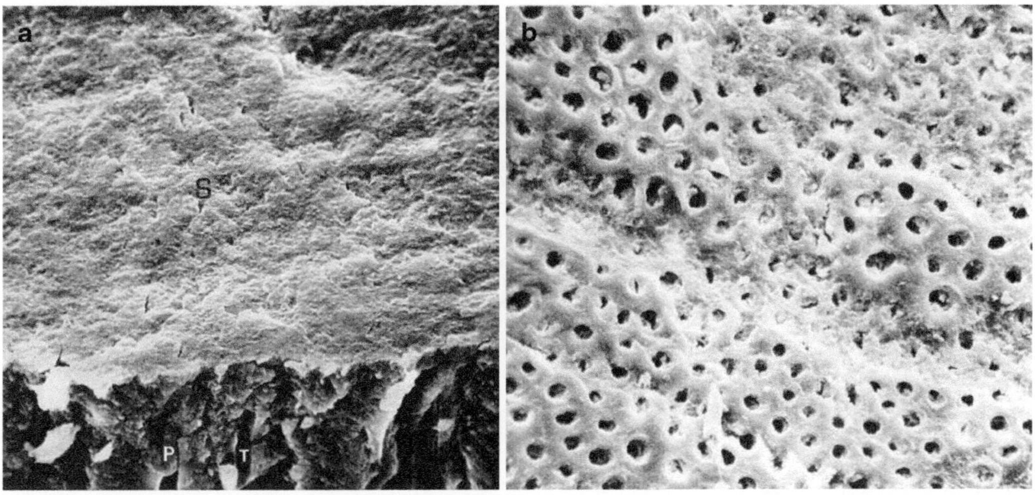

Fig. 2.6 (a, b) Brännström prepared shallow cavities in orthodontic premolars scheduled for extraction. The teeth were not restored but were left open to the oral cavity for up to 7 days. Sensitivity was scored immediately and after 1 week. The teeth were extracted and examined histologically and by SEM. On the left, the freshly prepared cavity dentin was covered with a smear layer. On the right, the smear layer dissolved from the exposed dentin after 1 week. Note how open are the tubules (From Figs. 14 and 15, Brännström (1981), with permission)

(Fig. 2.6a). He tested the initial sensitivity of the exposed dentin to air blasts and tactile probing and recorded their pain responses. He left the drilled cavities unfilled and exposed to saliva and oral bacteria. One week later, he had them return for rescoring of dentin sensitivity (Fig. 2.6b). He found that sensitivity had increased a great deal due, in part, to the loss of the smear layer. When the teeth were extracted for orthodontic treatment, and the pulps were examined histologically, he found that the pulpal surface of cut, exposed tubules that were allowed to dry in air, showed aspiration of some odontoblast nuclei into tubules. When dentin was exposed to saliva for a week, the pulps became infiltrated with acute inflammatory cells (Figs. 2.7a, b).

We now know that the ground dentin was covered by a smear layer that became covered with bacterial plaque within days. This biofilm created sufficient lactic acid to dissolve the smear layer and smear plugs (Kerns et al. 1991) within 1 week so that the dentin tubules would become hyperconductive. Thus, their increased dentin sensitivity was due, in part, to hyperconductive dentin (Brännström 1962).

2.6 Dynamics of Smear Layer Loss and Tubule Occlusion

Many dentists ask "how long do smear layers last on planed root surfaces?" Others ask how long it takes acid-etched dentinal tubules to close by remineralization. The answer to both of these questions is "about 1–2 weeks." In a now classic paper (Kerns et al. 1991), we used teeth extracted for periodontal reasons. Their cervical regions were root planed (Fig. 2.8a) and then divided into multiple slabs (2×3×1 mm): one served as a smear layer-covered control; another served as an EDTA-etched control with open tubules; another EDTA-etched specimen was treated with 3 % monopotassium-monohydrogen oxalate (pH 2.4) for 2 min to occlude the open tubules with crystals of calcium oxalate. Then the various dentin slabs were placed in denture flanges of denture patients for 1–4 weeks. At 1-week intervals, the dentin slabs were removed and processed for SEM.

Figure 2.8b shows dentin covered with a smear layer before it was placed in a denture flange. The image on the right shows a similar

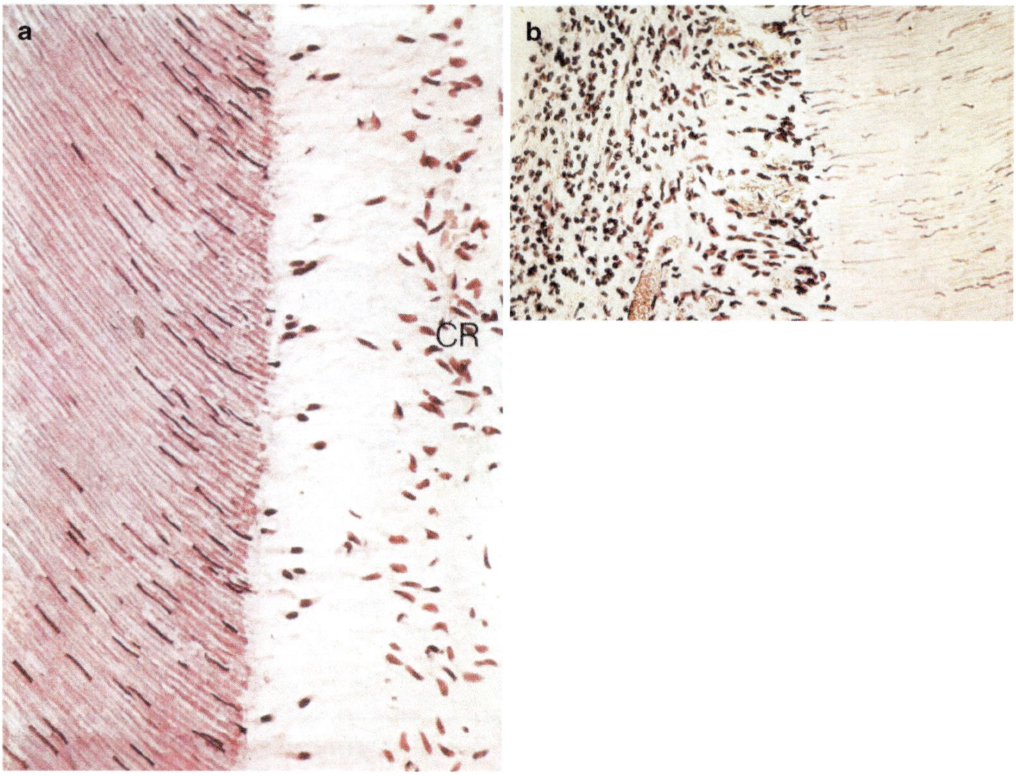

Fig. 2.7 (**a**) This tooth was allowed to air dry for 4 min and became painful after 20 s. Note the odontoblast layer has disappeared from beneath the dentin. Odontoblast nuclei are seen up inside the tubules, but no inflammation has occurred yet. One can easily identify the cell-free zone and the cell-rich (CR) zone (From Figs. 14 and 15, Brännström 1981, with permission). (**b**) This tooth's class V cavity was exposed to oral fluids for 1 week. The dentin was very painful. The pulp was heavily infiltrated with acute inflammatory cells. Pulpal capillaries were disrupted and venules were dilated (From Figs. 14 and 15, Brännström (1981), with permission)

sample that had been worn in the mouth for 1 week. Note that more than half the smear layer was lost and many open tubules were exposed. Figure 2.8c shows dentin treated with 18 % EDTA (pH 7) to remove the smear layer and expose open dentinal tubules. In the right panel is shown the appearance of similar dentin after 1 week where some of the tubules begin to be occluded by salivary salts. Fig. 2.8d show dentin that has remineralized for 2 weeks (left panel), while the right panel shows dentin that remineralized for 4 weeks. In Fig. 2.8e (left panel), dentin surfaces that were treated with 2.7 % acidic potassium oxalate for 1 min were covered with calcium oxalate crystals. In the right panel, similar dentin that had been in the mouth for 1 week showed loss of most of the calcium oxalate crystals and reappearance of some open tubules. However, some tubules remained occluded by calcium oxalate crystals below the surface.

Clinically, many patients do not complain of dentin hypersensitivity immediately after scaling and root planning (Fischer et al. 1991) but do so after 7–10 days. We believe that the lack of initial sensitivity is due to the smear layer created on root dentin by scaling; that then slowly dissolves over the next 7–10 days, making exposed dentinal tubules hyperconductive. If the patient remains untreated, these open sensitive dentinal tubules slowly begin to close by remineralization over the next 1–2 weeks. Thus, some patients may spontaneously heal but may be angry with their clinician. If patients who become hypersensitive in 7–10 days are then treated with 3 % potassium oxalate (BisBlock, Bisco Dental, Chicago, IL; SuperSeal, Phoenix, Fenton, Michigan; RemeSense), then

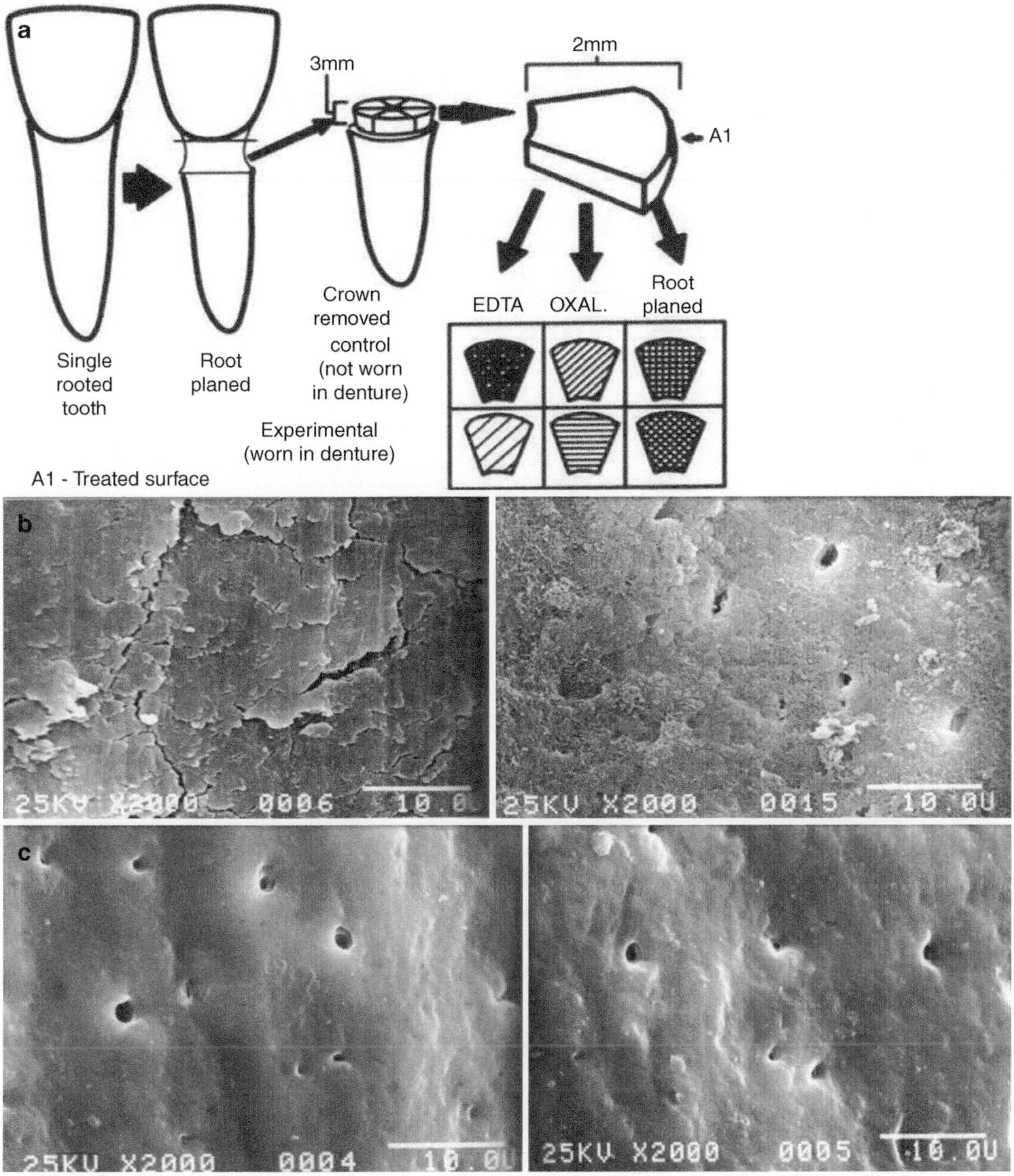

Fig. 2.8 (**a**–**e**) Kerns et al. (1991) placed dentin chips on denture flanges that were followed for up to several weeks. (**b**) Shows smear layer-covered dentin on the left. After 1 week, more than half the smear layer dissolved (*right*) opening many tubules. (**c**) If tubules were first opened with 18 % EDTA (*left*) and then exposed to saliva for a week, the tubules began to close by deposition of salivary mineral (*right*), which became more mineralized by 2 weeks more so (**d**, *left*) and more so after 4 weeks (*right*). (**e**) Dentin surface is covered with calcium oxalate crystals (*left*). After 1 week in the mouth, most of the calcium oxalate crystals on the dentin surface dissolved (*right*) (Kerns et al. (1991) with permission from the American Academy of Periodontology)

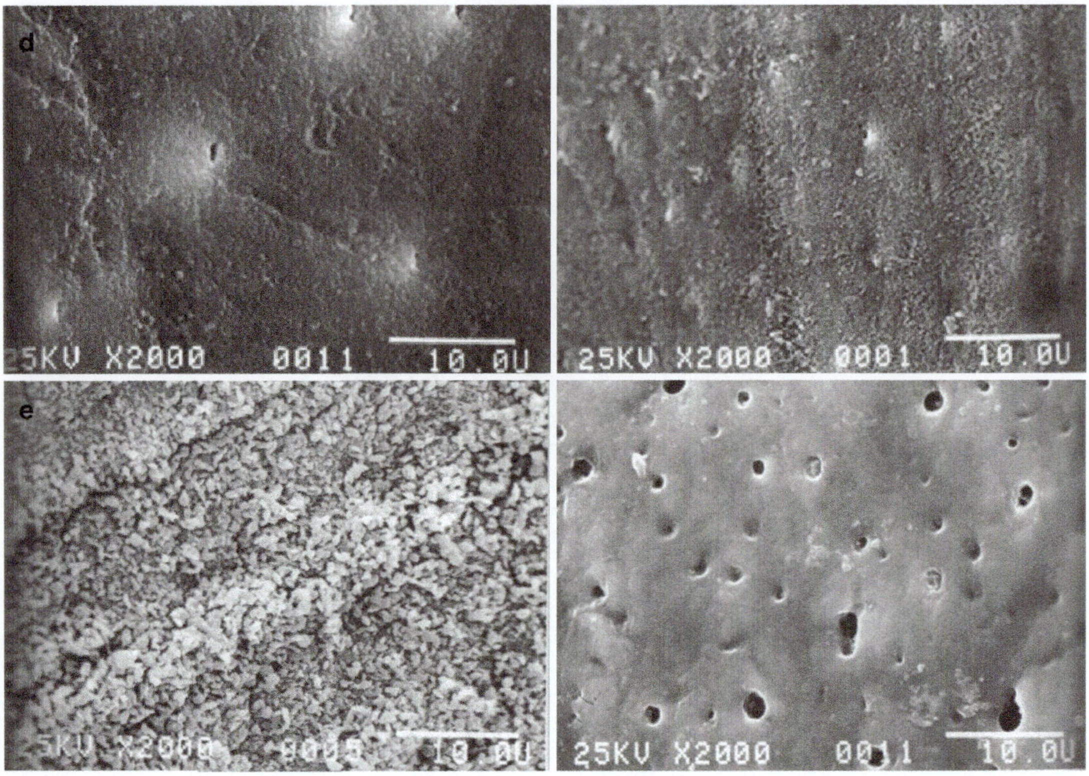

Fig. 2.8 (continued)

those open tubules can be closed temporarily with calcium oxalate crystals. An alternative to these professionally applied topical oxalates is the new potassium oxalate-containing desensitizing Listerine mouthwash called Listerine Advanced Defence Sensitive (LADS) (Fig. 2.9). This is only available in England but should be available in the USA this summer.

Remineralization of open dentinal tubules assumes that the patient has effective plaque control. If excessive plaque is frequently fed with fermentable carbohydrates, the plaque-derived lactic acid will etch away any attempts to remineralize. Patients who suffer from xerostomia do not have sufficient saliva to remineralize dentin.

2.7 Spontaneous Healing Mechanisms

The success of Brännström's (1962) use of oral fluids to induce pulpal inflammation under exposed, intact dentin encouraged Lundy and Stanley (1969) to repeat this experiment on a much wider range of patient ages (28–54 years), and to correlate their pain responses with pulpal histopathology over much longer times. Those authors recruited adult patients with asymptomatic teeth that were scheduled for extraction. Lundy and Stanley cut deep class V cavity preparations in those teeth under local anesthesia. The empty cavities were left exposed to saliva for 1–120 days. Just before extracting the teeth, the authors exposed these teeth to air blasts, probing, hot and cold stimuli, electric pulp testing, etc. and recorded the results. The teeth were then extracted and processed for light microscopy. When the authors correlated their clinical pain tests with the corresponding histopathologic results, they found that dentin sensitivity to air blasts and probing increased profoundly during the first week. The authors said that "it was quite evident that the degree of dentin sensitivity became very profound in the first week, sometimes becoming intolerable" (Table 2.1). The teeth with hypersensitive dentin were associated

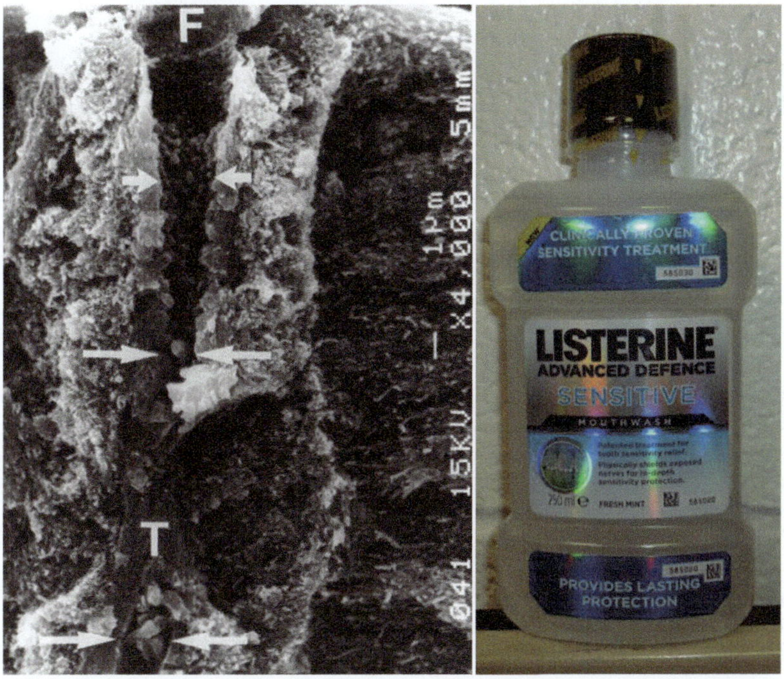

Fig. 2.9 A dentin disk with open tubules was treated with listerine advanced defence sensitive (LADS) desensitizing mouthrinse containing 1.4 wt % potassium oxalate (pH 4.2) twice a day for 60 s, for 1 week. The disk was then fractured to permit examination of intratubular contents below the surface. This scanning electron micrograph shows a funneled tubule orifice of a dentinal tubule. Acid-etching, used to open the tubule of smear layer debris removed the hypermineralized peritubular dentin matrix from the top 3–4 μm of the tubule. When treated with soluble potassium oxalate (KOx) in Listerine, the KOx diffused down the tubule until it could interact with intact peritubular dentin. The acidic (pH 4.2) mouthrinse liberated ionized calcium from the peritubular matrix, that reacted with the soluble KOx to form insoluble crystals of calcium oxalate (*double white arrows*). *T* indicates the continuation of the tubule lumen. When dentin fractures, the fracture plane is not always straight. The tubule lumen disappeared between the opposing white arrows and the region below the *T*. Note that the calcium oxalate crystals become larger the deeper they penetrate down the lumen. (Sharma et al. 2013, with permission)

Table 2.1 Histopathologic pulpal reactions in teeth with open cavities

	Less than 12 days	Over 12 days
Number of specimens[a]	26	22
Average postoperative time interval	5.0	84.0
(days)	(1–11 days)	(25–240 days)
Average age of patients	41.1	42.0
Average tooth size (code)[8]	3.4	3.0
Average remaining dentine thickness (mm)	0.9	1.2
Average degree of displacement	1.9	0.6
Average degree of superficial response	2.2	0.5
Average degree of deep response	2.5	0.8

[a]For these computations, those specimens that presented preoperatively formed irregular dentine were not included. From Lundy and Stanley (1969)

with acute inflammatory cells on their pulpal terminations of only the cut tubules. However, the subjective symptoms and histologic reactions were completely different at longer time periods (e.g., >12 days). The patients no longer complained of sensitivity to hot and cold food and drink even though the cavities remained open.

Bergenholz and Lindhe (1975) were intrigued by the possibility that bacterial plaque on dentin could cause pulpal inflammation. They prepared

Table 2.2 Histological response of monkey pulps to place extracts for 8 h (monkey 1) or 30 days (monkeys 2 and 3)

		Monkey 1		Monkey 2		Monkey 3	
		Test	Control	Test	Control	Test	Control
Mean remaining dentin thickness ± s.d. (mm)		1.1 ± 0.5	0.8 ± 0.4	1.0 ± 0.5	0.9 ± 0.5	1.1 ± 0.3	1.0 ± 0.2
Degree vascular labeling	0	0	4	8	7	2	5
	1	0	1	0	1	4	0
	2	6	1	0	0	0	0
	P-value	$P<0.01$		$P>0.1$		$P>0.01$	
Degree cell infiltration	0	5	5	2	6	0	4
	1	0	0	3	2	5	1
	2	1	1	3	0	1	0
	P-value	$P>0.1$		$0.05<P>0.1$		$P<0.05$	

Bergenholtz and Lindhe (1975) tested effects of water-soluble plaque extracts applied to exposed dentin for 8 h (monkey #1) or 30 days (monkeys 2 and 3). Each monkey received intravascular injection of colloidal carbon to label pulpal blood vessels just before sacrifice. Note high vascular labeling in monkey 1 and high leukocyte cell infiltration in pulps of monkeys 2 and 3

class V cavities in the cervical root dentin of monkeys. Then an extract of human dental plaque were sealed in the test cavity for 32 h causing the accumulation of bacterial plaque on those surfaces. After 32 h, they sacrificed the first monkey and examined the pulps by light microscopy. Those teeth treated with plaque extract exhibited pulpal inflammation, while control teeth treated with sterile buffer had no signs of pulpal inflammation (Bergenholz and Lindhe 1978). They also cut deep class V cavities in monkeys and then applied pooled human supragingival plaque extract to dentin every 5 min for 8 h (Table 2.2). Even water extracts free of bacteria caused pulpal inflammation under intact root dentin (Bergenholz 1981).

We believe that the works of Brännström (1962), Lundy and Stanley (1969), and Bergenholz (1977, 1981) provide the rationale for why patients with exposed cervical dentin show less dentin hypersensitivity if they maintain good plaque removal habits (Drisko 2007).

They showed that freshly exposed dentin is sensitive, but not hypersensitive. It becomes hypersensitive when bacterial products from septic saliva or bacterial plaque diffuse down exposed dentinal tubules and induce localized pulpal inflammation beneath the exposed tubules. Inflammation induces nerve sprouting, upregulation of a new class of sodium channels, and elevations in pulpal tissue pressure. These changes, combined with the loss of smear layers over the initial 5–7 days, cause an elevation in baseline outward fluid flow that is sufficient to bring intradental nerves closer to their activation thresholds, allowing previously innocuous hydrodynamic stimuli to cause severe pain.

Although Lundy and Stanley (1969) did not say it in their classic paper, Stanley later concluded that because there was no irritation dentin formation in the severely inflamed pulps, the disappearance of symptoms in the unfilled cavities over 12–90 days must have been due to decreases in dentin permeability that had no histologic correlates.

2.8 Spontaneously Healing of Hypersensitive Dentin

To investigate this possibility, Pashley et al. (1984a) cut class V cavities in the molar teeth of anesthetized dogs. They measured the permeability of the cavity dentin every hour for 6–8 h. They were surprised to find that in dogs with vital pulps, the permeability of the dentin fell about 15 % per hour for 6–8 h (Fig. 2.10). This was done under isolation so that neither saliva nor bacteria could touch the dentin. When pulpotomies were done in teeth before preparing the cavities, the permeability of the teeth did not decrease at all but increased over time. This confirmed that vital pulps somehow could decrease the permeability of dentin over time.

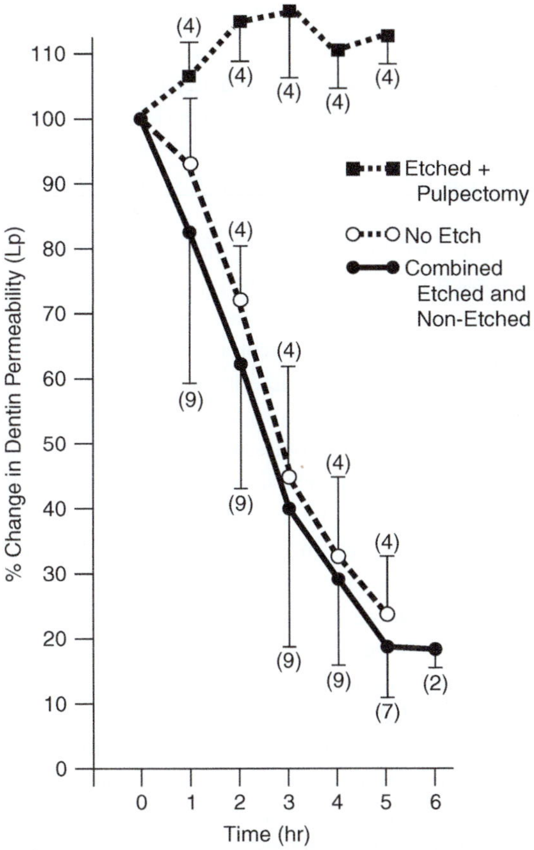

Fig. 2.10 Dentin permeability was measured in dog molars every hr for 6 h after preparing and acid-etching class V cavities. The *dotted line* shows results obtained in nonvital (pulpotomized) teeth. In those teeth, permeability increased over time. The *solid line* shows a 15 % decrease in dentin permeability each hr for 6 h. Each value is mean of number of teeth shown in parentheses ± 1 SD (From Pashley et al. (1984b), with permission)

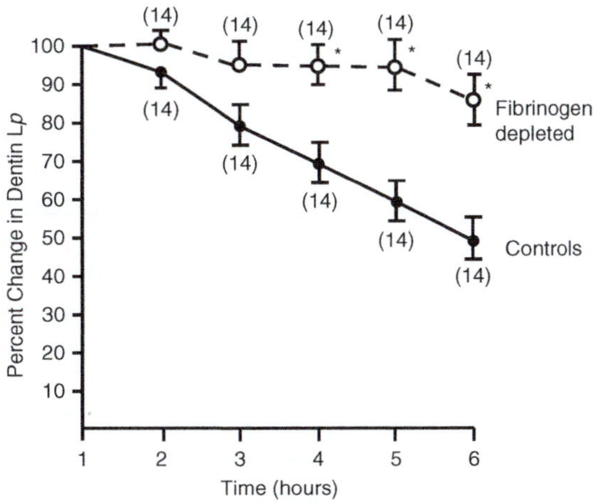

Fig. 2.11 Changes in dentin permeability of dog dentin in vivo over time. The *solid lines* are data obtained from control dogs over 6 h. The *dotted lines* indicate results obtained in dogs that were depleted of all of their plasma fibrinogen before the experiment began. Apparently, fibrinogen and other large plasma proteins leak out of irritated pulpal capillaries and partially occlude dentinal tubules over time (From Pashley et al. (1984a), with permission)

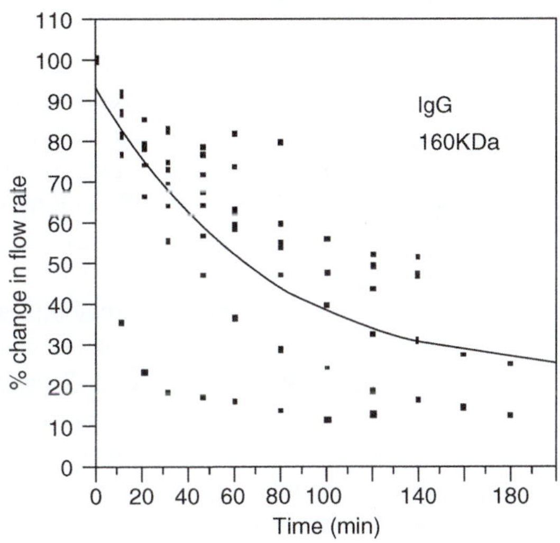

Fig. 2.12 Decrease in dentin permeability in vitro when dilute IgG (100 μg/ml) was filtered from pulp side of dentin to occlusal side for 3 h (From Hahn and Overton 1997 with permission)

Apparently pulpal irritation by cavity preparation and fluid filtration induces pulpal inflammation that increases the permeability of pulpal capillaries and venules to plasma proteins. In the patients of Lundy and Stanley (1969), this outward leakage of plasma proteins may have stopped the inward diffusion of salivary solutions of bacterial products, allowing the pulps to undergo healing even though the dentin remained exposed. When Pashley et al. (1984a) depleted dogs of fibrinogen in vivo prior to cutting cavities into dentin, the decrease in dentin permeability over time was greatly reduced (Fig. 2.11). Large plasma proteins like fibrinogen and immunoglobulins (Fig. 2.12) leak out of these vessels and adsorb to the walls of the tubules where they partially occlude them.

Thus, the pulpodentin complex is not a passive set of structures but is a vital, dynamic complex that reacts to external trauma by a series of events designed to protect the pulp from external threats.

The inflammatory mediators that are released during pulpal inflammation include histamine, bradykinin, prostaglandins, and complement. The inflammatory mediators sensitize pulpal nerves and increase local pulpal blood flow and local tissue pressure, causing an increase in outward fluid flow, much like the well-documented increase in outward gingival fluid flow that is seen in inflamed gingival tissues (Pashley 1976). If this increase in outward fluid flow approaches the critical outward fluid velocity reported by Charoehlaro et al. (2007) of 5.8 nL/s mm^2, the A-δ nociceptors beneath that exposed dentin might become "hypersensitive" to hydrodynamic stimuli relative to their preinflammed sensitivity.

2.9 Clinical Considerations: Methods of Dentin Sensitization

We speculate that during periodontal surgery, roots are planed free of calculus, inadvertently removing cementum and exposing cervical dentinal tubules. The newly exposed dentin is covered by a smear layer generated by curettes. Over a period of 5–10 days, this surface becomes colorized by multiple species of oral bacteria to form a biofilm. As this biofilm metabolizes ingested sucrose, it produces sufficient organic acids to remove the smear layer over 5–7 days and make that dentin both hyperconductive and more sensitive. The loss of the smear layer increases the permeability (Kerns et al. 1991) of dentin to bacterial products (Ferraz et al., 2011), causing pulpal inflammation that makes pulpal nerves hypersensitive. This localized pulpal inflammation increases capillary permeability to plasma proteins including immunoglobulins, fibrinogen, and albumin; these molecules diffuse into dentinal tubules and adsorb to the tubule walls causing decreases in dentin permeability (Pashley et al. 1981, 1984a, 1985) over the next 7–8 days. This allows the transient dentin hypersensitivity to spontaneously resolve without any treatment. However, in a minority of patients, this spontaneous resolution does not occur and these patients remain hypersensitive. The mechanism of this prolonged hypersensitivity is unknown. Perhaps these patients have experienced multiple episodes of pulpal inflammation that have healed by scar formation causing a loss of pulpal capillaries near dentin. The lack of local capillaries might prevent leakage of plasma proteins into exposed dentin. Alternatively, patients may generate too much outward dentinal fluid flow that flushes these plasma proteins from the tubules preventing tubule occlusion. Such patients need to be treated with a topical tubule occlusion agent (Gluma or potassium oxalate-containing products like SuperSeal or Listerine Advanced Defence Sensitive) to reverse their hypersensitivity. Tubule occlusion lowers the inward diffusion of bacterial products, allowing resolution of local pulpal inflammation, reversing nerve sprouting, allowing fewer more sensitive sodium channels (Na_v 1.8 and 1.9) to be expressed in pulpal nerves, and decreasing dentin sensitivity. In this scheme, bacterial products and pulpal inflammation must be controlled if we are to prevent the development of dentin hypersensitivity.

Future occluding treatments for dentin sensitivity should include antimicrobial agents (Sharma et al. 2004; Charles et al. 2013) and anti-inflammatory agents that can all act in concert to prevent the development of localized pulpal inflammation beneath open, sensitive dentinal tubules.

Acknowledgement This work was supported, in part, by R01 DE015306 from the NIDCR to DHP (PI) and by the King Abdulazziz University School of Dentistry to Prof. Pashley as their Hi-Ci dental scholar.

References

Bergenholz G (1977) Effect of bacterial products on inflammatory reactions in the dental pulp. Scand J Dent Res 85:122–129

Bergenholz G (1981) Inflammatory response of the dental pulp to bacterial irritation. J Endod 7:100–104

Bergenholz G, Lindhe J (1975) Effect of soluble plaque factors on inflammatory reactions in the dental pulp. Scand J Dent Res 83:153–158

Bergenholz G, Lindhe J (1978) Effect of experimentally induced marginal periodontitis and periodontal scaling on the dental pulp. J Clin Periodontal 5:59–73

Berggren E, Heyeraas KJ (1999) The role of sensory neuropeptides and nitric oxide on pulpal blood flow and tissue pressure in the ferret. J Dent Res 78:1535–1543

Brännström M (1962) The elicitation of pain in human dentine and pulp by chemical stimuli. Arch Oral Biol 7:59–62

Brännström M (1981) Dentin and pulp in restorative dentistry, 1st edn. Dental Therapeutics AB, Nacka, p 17, 20, 21

Brännström M (1992) Etiology of dentin hypersensitivity. Proc Finn Dent Soc 88(Suppl 1):7–13

Byers M, Närhi MVO (1999) Dental injury models: experimental tools for understanding neuroinflammatory nociceptor functions. Crit Rev Oral Biol Med 10:4–39

Byers M, Henry MA, Närhi MVO (2012) Chapter 7. Dental innervation and its response to tooth injury. In: Hargreaves KM, Goodis HE, Tay FR (eds) Dental pulp. Quintessence Publishing Co. Inc, Chicago, pp 133–157

Charles CA, McGuire JA, Qaquish J, Amini P (2013) Increasing antiplaque/antigingivitis of an essential oil-containing mouthrinse over time: an in vivo study. Gen Dent 61:23–28

Charoenlarp P, Wanachantararak S, Vongsavan N, Matthews B (2007) Pain and the rate of dentinal fluid flow produced by hydrostatic pressure stimulation of exposed dentin in man. Arch Oral Biol 52:625–631.

Ciucchi B, Bouillaguet S, Holz J, Pashley DH (1995) Dentinal fluid dynamics in human teeth, in vivo. J Endod 21:191–194

Drisko C (2007) Oral hygiene and periodontal considerations in preventing and managing dentine hypersensitivity. Int Dent J 57:399–410

Ferraz CC, Henry MA, Hargreaves KM, Diogenes A (2011) Lipopolysaccharide from Porphyromonas gingivalis sensitizes capsaicin-sensitive nociceptors. J Endod 37:45–48

Fischer C, Wennberg A, Fischer RG, Attström R (1991) Clinical evaluation of pulp and dentine sensitivity after supragingival and subgingival scaling. Endod Dent Traumatol 7:259–265

Fouad AF (2012) Chapter 11. Molecular mediators of pulpal inflammation. In: Hargreaves KM, Goodis HE, Tay FR (eds) Seltzer and Bender's dental pulp, 2nd edn. Quintessence Publishing Co., Inc, Chicago, pp 241–275

Hahn C-L, Overton B (1997) The effects of immunoglobulins on the convective permeability of human dentine in vitro. Arch Oral Biol 42:835–843

Henry MA, Luo S, Foley BD, Rzasa RS, Johnson LR, Levinson SR (2009) Sodium channel expression and localization at demyelinated sites in painful human dental pulp. J Pain 10:750–758

Heyeraas KJ, Kvinnsland I (1992) Tissue pressure and blood flow in pulpal inflammation. Proc Finn Dent Soc 88(Suppl 1):393–401

Kerns DG, Scheidt MJ, Pashley DH, Horner JA, Strong SL, Van Dyke TE (1991) Dentinal tubule occlusion and root hypersensitivity. J Periodontol 62:421–428

Lundy T, Stanley HR (1969) Correlation of pulpal histopathology and clinical symptoms in human teeth subjected to experimental irritation. Oral Surg Oral Med Oral Pathol 27:187–201

Luo A, Perry GM, Levison SR, Henry MA (2008) Na_v 1.7 expression is increased in painful human dental pulp. Mol Pain 4:16

Matthews B, Vongsavan N (1994) Interactions between neural and hydrodynamic mechanisms in dentine and pulp. Arch Oral Biol 39(Suppl):87S–95S

Närhi M, Jyvasjarv E, Vitanen A, Huopaniemi T, Ngassapa D, Hirvonen T (1992) Role of intradental A and C type nerve fibers in dental pain mechanisms. Proc Finn Dent Soc 8(Suppl 1):507–516

Nissan R, Segal H, Pashley DH, Stevens R, Trowbridge H (1995) Ability of bacterial endotoxin to diffuse through human dentin. J Endod 21:62–64

Pashley DH (1976) A mechanistic analysis of gingival fluid production. J Periodontol Res 11:121–134

Pashley DH (1985) Dentin-predentin complex and its permeability. Physiological overview. J Dent Res 64(Spec Iss):613–620

Pashley DH (1992) Mechanistic analysis of fluid distribution across the pulpodentin complex. J Endod 18:72–75

Pashley DH, Matthews WG (1993) The effects of outward forced convective flow on inward diffusion in human dentine, in vitro. Arch Oral Biol 38:577–582

Pashley DH, Tay FR (2012) Pulpodentin complex. In: Hargreaves KM, Goodis HE, Tay FR (eds) Seltzer and Bender's Dental Pulp, 2nd edn. Quitessence Publishing Co. Inc., Chicago, pp. 47–65

Pashley DH, Nelson R, Pashley EL (1981) In vivo fluid movement across dentin in the dog. Arch Oral Biol 26:707–710

Pashley DH, Galloway SE, Stewart FP (1984a) Effects of fibrinogen in vivo on dentin permeability in the dog. Arch Oral Biol 29:725–728

Pashley DH, Kepler EE, Williams EC, O'Meara JA (1984b) The effect on dentine permeability of time following cavity preparation in days. Arch Oral Biol 29:65–68

Puapichartdumcong P, Ikeda H, Suda H (2005) Outward fluid flow reduces inward diffusion of bacterial lipopolysaccharide across intact and demineralized dentine. Arch Oral Biol 50:707–713

Renton T, Yiangou Y, Plumpton C, Tate S, Bountra C, Anand P (2005) Sodium channel Na_v 1.8 immunoreactivity in painful human dental pulp. BMC Oral Health 5:5

Sharma N et al (2004) Adjunctive benefit of an essential oil-containing mouthrinse in reducing plaque and gingivitis in patients who brush and floss regularly. J Am Dent Assoc 135:496–504

Sharma D, Hong CX, Heipp PS (2013) A novel potassium oxalate-containing tooth-desensitizing mouthrinse: A comparative in vitro study. J Dent 41:S4;S18–S27

Ten Cate AR (1998) Chapter 9. In: Oral histology development structure and function., p 191

Vongsavan N, Matthews B (1992) Fluid flow through cat dentine in vivo. Arch Oral Biol 37:175–185

Warren CA, Mok L, Gordon S, Fouad AF, Gold MS (2008) Quantitation of neural protein in extirpated tooth pulp. J Endod 34:7–10

Wells JE, Bingham V, Rowland KC, Hatton J (2007) Expression of Na_v 1.9 channels in human dental pulp and trigeminal ganglion. J Endod 33:1172–1176

Etiology and Predisposing Factors to Dentin Hypersensitivity

3

Mohanad Al-Sabbagh

Abstract

Dentin hypersensitivity is a prevalent and common complaint in dentistry. Identification of the etiological and predisposing factors for dentin hypersensitivity is of prime importance in the diagnosis and treatment planning of this dental complaint. In order to have a clinical manifestation of dentin hypersensitivity, the dentin must be exposed to the oral environment. Dentin exposure results from one or more etiological factors that lead to loss of enamel and/or loss of cementum and overlaying periodontal tissues. Many dental and medical conditions have been linked to dentin hypersensitivity as etiological or predisposing factors. Some periodontal or restorative treatment may initiate the dentin hypersensitivity symptoms. In this chapter, we will shed light on all the etiological and contributory factors responsible for dentin hypersensitivity.

3.1 Introduction

Pain elicited by the application of external stimuli to exposed dentin in the oral cavity is a common symptom among the adult population. Dentin hypersensitivity (DH) is often self-reported by patients and is described clinically as an exaggerated pain response to external stimuli such as cold or hot beverages and toothbrushing. In most cases, the pain response is initiated and persists only during the application of stimulus to exposed dentin. This condition can affect the patient's day-to-day activities such as eating, drinking, toothbrushing, and, occasionally, breathing. DH may present either as a chronic condition causing minor discomfort or low-level pain or as an acute condition causing severe debilitating pain requiring immediate care (Curro 1990). Johnson and colleagues mentioned DH as an enigma because it is routinely encountered but not well understood (Johnson et al. 1982). It has recently been reported that one in eight patients from general dental practices in the northwest USA were affected by DH (Cunha-Cruz et al. 2013). Furthermore, the incidence of DH tends to increase with an increase in the tooth wear and with increased retention of natural dentition that is susceptible to gingival recession (Al-Sabbagh

M. Al-Sabbagh, DDS, MS
Division of Periodontology,
Department of Oral Health Practice,
University of Kentucky College of Dentistry,
D-438, 800 Rose Street, Lexington, KY 40536, USA
e-mail: malsa2@email.uky.edu

S. Taha, B.H. Clarkson (eds.), *Clinician's Guide to the Diagnosis and Management of Tooth Sensitivity*,
DOI 10.1007/978-3-642-45164-5_3, © Springer-Verlag Berlin Heidelberg 2014

et al. 2004). Therefore, oral health practitioners must perform careful screening, obtain a differential diagnosis, and provide effective treatment.

3.2 Concept of Dentin Hypersensitivity

Dentin is a mineralized connective tissue of the tooth that is covered by enamel or cementum. It consists of numerous channels called dentinal tubules that contain odontoblastic processes projecting from the odontoblast cells present on the outer surface of the dentinal pulp. The dentinal tubule also contains nerve terminals and fluid. In 1962, Brannstorm and Astrom proposed the "hydrodynamic theory" as an explanation of DH (Brannstrom 1986). This theory suggests that upon stimulus, the fluid in the dentinal tubule undergoes rapid movement that can either damage odontoblast cell or activate the nerve terminals to cause pain. Myelinated A fiber is responsible for the perception of pain in DH. A transmission electron microscopy (TEM) study of hypersensitive human radicular dentin demonstrated wide and empty dentinal tubules in comparison to desensitized dentin that appears to be occluded with radiopaque materials (Yoshiyama et al. 1990). Absi et al. reported that, compared with nonsensitive teeth, hypersensitive teeth contain eight times more dentinal tubules and that these tubules are twice as wide (Absi et al. 1987). These findings appear consistent with the hydrodynamic theory. The larger number of open and wider dentinal tubules exposed in the oral environment will ultimately result in increased fluid movement upon external stimulus and will subsequently increase the pain response. Furthermore, the mechanism of action of several available DH treatments that target or occlude or narrow the exposed dentinal tubules can be explained by the hydrodynamic theory.

3.3 Etiology of Dentin Hypersensitivity

The loss of tooth structure and the exposure of dentin to the oral cavity is a requisite mechanism for the development of the clinical symptoms of DH. The process involving the loss of enamel and/or cementum and of the overlying periodontal attachment apparatus plays an important role in exposing dentin in the oral environment. This process is "lesion localization" and is one phase in the development of DH (Dababneh et al. 1999). After exposure, the patent dentinal tubules remain wide open and thus are predisposed to any stimulus, called the phase of "lesion initiation." However, not all exposed dentin is sensitive (Rimondini et al. 1995). This incongruity can be explained by the deposition of the smear layer that can occlude the dentinal tubules, rendering them nonsensitive (Brannstrom and Garberoglio 1980). On the other hand, lesion initiation can be achieved by the process of abrasion, erosion, and gingival recession, which can result in the loss of tooth structure and the exposure of dentin. Although not all exposed dentin is sensitive, exposed dentin can be sensitive if it possesses patent dentinal tubules (Brannstrom 1965). A number of etiological and predisposing factors may expose dentin to the oral cavity by causing the loss of enamel and/or periodontal supporting tissue, thereby resulting in DH. A summary of the etiological factors contributing to DH is represented in Fig. 3.1.

3.3.1 Loss of Enamel

3.3.1.1 Attrition

Attrition is defined as the gradual loss of tooth substance because of occlusal contacts with opposing dentition or restoration without the presence of food (Hattab and Yassin 2000; Kaidonis 2008). Physiological attrition gradually increases with age and accompanies the reduction of cusp height and the occlusal incline plane, with the loss of enamel and dentin (Hattab and Yassin 2000). However, it is interesting to note that the loss of dental hard tissue may not be a symptom of DH because of the formation of secondary dentin (Johnson and Sivers 1987; Hattab and Yassin 2000). Although attrition is a physiologic process, it can be accelerated by other factors, such as parafunctional habits, clenching and bruxism, traumatic occlusion, grinding, and malocclusion (Hattab and Yassin 2000). The occlusal and incisal surfaces are primarily affected, and tooth wear can be extensive in severe bruxism

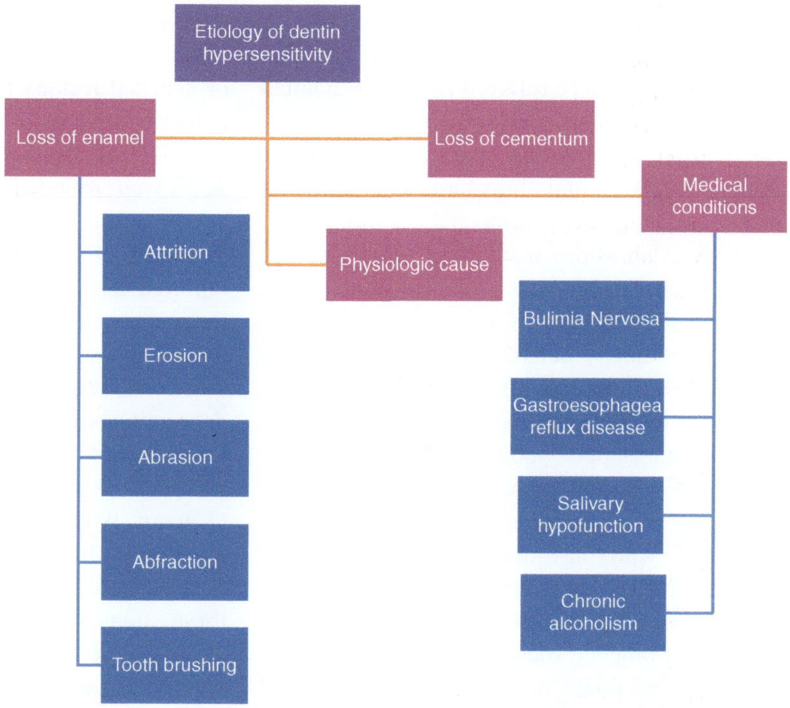

Fig. 3.1 Flow chart of the etiological factors contributing to DH

(Litonjua et al. 2003a). It may also involve the interproximal surfaces of the tooth, where tooth wear is associated with a decrease in the dental arch (Murphy 1964; Grippo et al. 2004). Studies have reported that bruxism may affect 8–20 % of the adult population (Glaros 1981), and tooth wear progresses more rapidly in patients with bruxism than in those with no bruxism (Xhonga 1977). Smith and associates reported that bruxism alone is an etiological factor in 11 % of referred cases of tooth wear and was the contributing etiological factor in approximately two-thirds of cases (Smith and Knight 1984). The clinical feature of attrition is characterized by an area with a relatively flat facet accompanying a well-circumscribed border on the cusp tip or ridge of a molar or the incisal edge of the anterior teeth (Litonjua et al. 2003a; Hattab and Yassin 2000). In the opposing arch, similar facets can be appreciated clinically. In areas in which dentin is exposed, the lesion appears to be flat without "cupping or scooping" (Kaidonis 2008). Although attrition can act independently, several combinations of the mechanism of tooth wear could act synergistically, thereby affecting the progression of loss of dental hard tissue. These combined mechanisms of tooth wear consist of "attrition-abfraction" and "attrition-corrosion," which involves the *integrated action* of stress and corrosive agents on the areas of tooth wear because of attrition (Grippo et al. 2004). In summary, attrition can be exaggerated by parafunctional habits such as bruxism and by other predisposing factors such as abrasion, erosion, and abfraction, which result in the progressive loss of dental hard tissue and exposure of the dentin (Fig. 3.2).

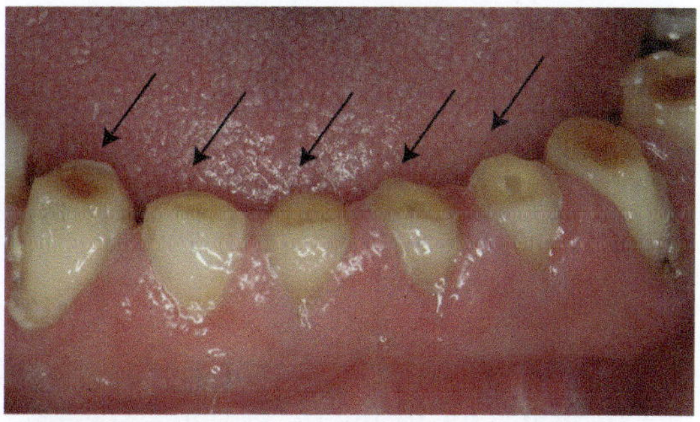

Fig. 3.2 An elderly patient suffered from attrition due to gradual physiological loss of occlusal tooth substance

3.3.1.2 Abrasion

Dental abrasion is the pathologic wearing of teeth as the result of abnormal processes, habits, or abrasive substances. It is a non-carious loss of tooth substance that is deprived of bacterial involvement. It can be referred to as a mechanical process that produces tooth wear because of friction caused by external materials or objects (Knight 1969). Dental abrasion has been associated with diet, occupation, and toothbrushing. Mechanical abrasions result from the consumption of a coarse diet that produces wear on the tooth surface. This type of tooth wear is relatively common clinically but is frequently overlooked (Grippo et al. 2004). It often involves the buccal surface of the lower molars and the palatal surfaces of the upper molars (Kaidonis 2008). Certain occupations can result in dental abrasion; frequently affected are carpenters, tailors, and musicians, who may demonstrate abrasion of maxillary incisal edges (Hattab and Yassin 2000; Johnson and Sivers 1987). Other activities involving foreign objects, such as biting pens or hairpins, smoking pipes, or biting one's nails could result in the development of notched abrasive lesions on the incisal edges. The clinical presentation of abrasive lesions appears to involve the entire occlusal surface, unlike attrition, which affects the wear facet. The exposed dentin appears to be scooped (Kaidonis 2008). Abrasive lesions may have sharp margins, in contrast to the broad and smooth margins of erosive lesions (Levitch et al. 1994). The most common cause of dental abrasion is toothbrushing. Toothbrush abrasion can result from incorrect technique, the application of heavy forces during brushing (Padbury and Ash 1974; Bergstrom and Lavstedt 1979), the frequency of toothbrushing (Phaneuf et al. 1962; Dyer et al. 2000; Bergstrom and Lavstedt 1979), bristle stiffness (Zimmer et al. 2011), and the use of abrasive toothpaste (Osborne-Smith et al. 1999; Dyer et al. 2000). The prevalence of toothbrushing as a causative factor is, however, unclear; published studies suggest that it affects 5–86 % of members of the population studied (Litonjua et al. 2003a). The cervical area at the cement-enamel junction on the buccal surface of all teeth is predominantly affected by toothbrush abrasion. The lesion appears as a V-shaped or rounded notch and commonly affects the maxillary canine, premolar, and first molar regions (Hattab and Yassin 2000; Bishop et al. 1997). Litonjua and co-workers studied the morphology of cervical lesions by analyzing experimentally induced toothbrush abrasive lesions. They found that 50 % of abrasive lesions were wedge shaped, 22 % were rounded, and 28 % of lesions were a combination of wedge shaped and round (Litonjua et al. 2004). Kitchin and colleagues reported an association between oral hygiene and the presence of abrasions: patients with good oral hygiene were more likely to exhibit abrasion than those with deprived oral hygiene. Also, the incidence of abrasion of the cementum and dentin increased from 42 % among patients aged 20–29 years to 76 % among those aged 50–59 years (Kitchin 1941). The dentin and cementum are less dense than enamel; therefore, tissue loss occurs more rapidly and progresses farther in these areas (Davis and Winter 1980). Right-handed patients exhibit more lesions on the teeth on the left side of the month than on those on the right side, probably because they use more force when brushing the left side of the mouth (Sangnes and Gjermo 1976). Radentz and associates reported that patients use more brushing force on the initial areas they brush; thus, these areas are more likely to suffer abrasion due to increased brushing forces (Radentz et al. 1976). Bergstrom and co-workers examined 818 individual adult groups and found a 30 % prevalence of cervical abrasion and a 12 % prevalence of wedge-shaped cervical lesions. They also reported a relationship between prevalence and severity of abrasion and the frequency of toothbrushing (patients who brushed twice daily), particularly when a horizontal toothbrushing technique was used (Bergstrom and Lavstedt 1979; Bartlett and Shah 2006). Although a relationship between the severity of abrasion and toothbrushing has been reported, some authors believe that erosion may play an important role in the progression of tooth wear. Attin and associates evaluated the period of remineralization of enamel previously eroded by brushing abrasion and concluded that the resistance to abrasion of eroded enamel continually increases as remineralization time increases (Attin et al. 2000). An in situ study by Jaeggi and colleagues was designed to assess the effect of

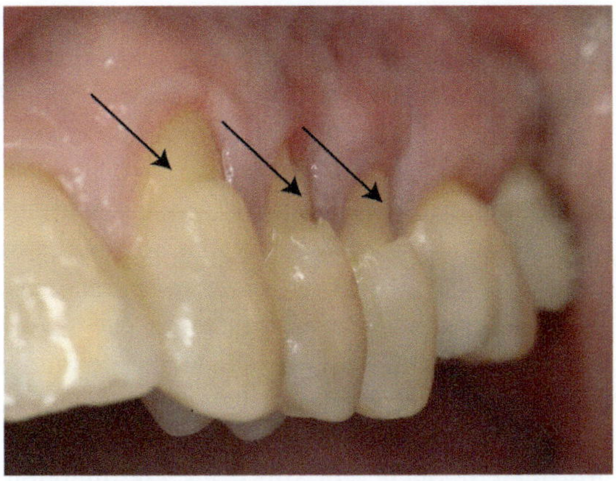

Fig. 3.3 Pathologic wearing of tooth substance of abrasion lesion (*arrows*) as the result of mechanical friction of foreign object

tooth bushing at 0, 30, and 60 min after the exposure of enamel to citric acid (an erosive agent). Toothbrush abrasion was more severe at 0 min than at 60 min; thus, it is recommended that patients avoid brushing for at least 1 h after the intake of acidic food or beverages to allow a period of remineralization that can reestablish the resistance of formerly eroded enamel to toothbrush abrasion (Jaeggi and Lussi 1999). Patients with partial dentures may show signs of abrasion because of the lesions caused by clasps. Grippo and co-workers suggested that, although abrasion can act independently to produce the loss of dental tissue, it can also occur in combination with other predisposing factors, such as attrition, erosion, and abfraction, to produce a more additive effect on the process of tooth wear (Grippo et al. 2004). When it occurs in combination with attrition or abfraction, abrasion can further exaggerate the loss of tooth structure by friction, heavy occlusal forces, and the accumulation of stress concentration by loading forces on the weaker areas, subsequently causing the tooth substance to break (Grippo et al. 2004) (Fig. 3.3).

3.3.1.3 Corrosion/Erosion

Dental erosion is the loss of mineralized dental hard tissue caused by the direct impact of exogenous and endogenous acids. These acids produce a chemical reaction leading to the dissolution of hydroxyapatite crystals and to the softening and eventual loss of dental hard tissue. The term "corrosion" has been encouraged as a replacement for "erosion" because it more precisely describes the chemical and electrochemical actions that can cause tooth wear (Grippo et al. 2004). The lesion can be self-reported by patients as an esthetic concern or may be associated with dentin hypersensitivity. Erosive lesions in their early stages may appear as smooth concave or rounded defects, whereas advanced erosive lesions may display concavities identified as cupping (Litonjua et al. 2003a). The clinical presentation of erosion can be easily differentiated from bacterial decay that produces rough lesions (Hattab and Yassin 2000). Erosion associated with extrinsic factors such as diet may manifest itself as a scooped-out depression on the labial surface of the maxillary front teeth (Hattab and Yassin 2000; Johnson and Sivers 1987; Litonjua et al. 2003a). Erosion can affect younger children. A recent survey reported that the prevalence of dental erosion was 15 % in children aged 12 years and was twice as high in those aged 15 years. Furthermore, the mandibular first molars were the most frequently affected by dental erosion (Arnadottir et al. 2010). Although erosion can basically affect any teeth in the mouth, the site and severity of the lesions may depend on the exposure and frequency of the erosive materials or agents that come into contact with the teeth. The dissolution of the tooth surface results from extrinsic or intrinsic acids. Exposure of the tooth to extrinsic acids can occur as the result of diet, medication, occupation, or environment. The most common source of dietary acid is liquid drinks such as grapefruit, lime, or orange juice or wine. Aerated drinks such as colas can produce erosive lesions. Acid is also present in pickled foods and citrus fruits. Beverages popular in the USA, such as sports drinks (Gatorade), energy drinks (Red Bull), aerated drinks (Mountain Dew and Coca-Cola), can erode both the enamel and the root (Ehlen et al. 2008). Holding the drink in the mouth for longer periods before swallowing and taking long sips has been associated with the risk of erosion (Johansson et al. 2004). It has also been suggested that drinking methods should be addressed in the dietary counseling of patients with dental erosion (Johansson et al. 2004). Grenby and colleagues reported that some "healthful drinks," such as pure citrus juice, exhibit higher dental erosive properties than carbonated cola drinks (Grenby et al. 1989). Commonly, exposed dentin surfaces may not be sensitive because of the natural process of occlusion of tubules by a smear layer. However, it is quite possible that the abrasive action of a toothbrush or even contact with erosive agents can eliminate the protective smear layer and expose the dentinal tubule, thereby creating a potentially sensitive site. Zandim and co-workers reported that several natural orange juices, such as those of navel oranges, Valencia oranges, and mandarin oranges, are more effective in exposing the dentinal tubules and removing the smear layer than are the juices of lime oranges and limes. However, when lime orange and lime juices were applied in combination with toothbrush friction, significantly more of the smear layer was removed (Zandim et al. 2008). Therefore, it has been suggested that erosive acids may be a predisposing factor in the progression of dentin tissue loss and sensitivity because it can act synergistically with abrasion in the oral cavity. A recent meta-analysis found that soft drinks are associated with a 2.4-fold higher risk of dental erosion (Li et al. 2012). Saliva and local fluid contribute protective functions that can help protect both enamel and dentin against the dental erosive process (Knight 1969). Properties of saliva, such as its cleansing, buffering capacity (Piangprach et al. 2009), remineralization, and acquired pellicle (Nekrashevych and Stosser 2003) can protect the tooth surface from acid attack. Piangprach and associates found that the concentrations of urea and salivary buffering capacity were higher in saliva samples of patients with erosive lesions than in samples from patients without erosion (Piangprach et al. 2009). Low saliva flow and poor buffering capacity allow the constant retention of exogenous and endogenous acids that would potentiate the erosive events on dental tissue (Zero and Lussi 2005). The critical pH of enamel is approximately 5.5; intermittent or continuous exposure of enamel to any acidic product with a pH lower than 5.5 can dissolve hydroxyapatite crystals (Meurman and ten Cate 1996). It has been reported that the pH of a cola-type drink is lower than this critical pH and is sufficient to demineralize the enamel (Ferrazzano et al. 2012a). However, it is interesting to note that once the tooth's contact with the acidic agent is stopped or a chelating material is provided, the process of demineralization ends. Because erosion is a multifactorial event, oral health providers should evaluate the condition and diagnose the etiology of the erosive lesion. Dentists should recommend that patients control their frequency of soft drink consumption, should educate them about the consequences if it is continued, and should provide replacements such as milk as a substitute to prevent the progression of dental erosion. Zero and co-workers have suggested that there is a strong connection between dentin hypersensitivity and erosion (Zero and Lussi 2005).

Some forms of erosion can be associated with occupation. Occupation erosion occurs as the result of workers' exposure to erosive agents over a long period of time. Petersen and colleagues screened workers in a German battery factory and reported severe erosion on the front teeth and attrition on the posterior teeth of those who were exposed to sulfuric acid (Petersen and Gormsen 1991). Gas-chlorinated swimming pools with water maintained at a pH of 2.7 generated dental erosion because of the exposure of the swimmers to acid (Centerwall et al. 1986). Gray and associates reported cervical erosion and occlusal pitting in patients whose occupation was associated with wine tasting (Gray et al. 1998). The severity of facial erosion of the maxillary front teeth was increased in patients employed in pharmaceutical and biotechnological work because of an increased exposure to proteolytic enzymes (Westergaard et al. 2001). Dental products may be associated with dental erosion because of either excessive toothbrushing or faulty oral hygiene practices. Some over-the-counter mouthwashes have a low pH because of their ethanol content and may have the potential to expose the dentinal tubule (Bhatti et al. 1994). An in vitro study has demonstrated the remineralization potential of fluoride toothpaste on erosive lesions

(Rirattanapong et al. 2012). Toothbrushing after consuming an acidic diet can speed up the chemical erosion activity on the tooth surface and may increase patients' susceptibility to dental erosion (Zero 1996; Jaeggi and Lussi 1999).

Another etiological factor for dental erosion is stomach acid, a key source of intrinsic acid. Stomach acid can enter the oral cavity as a consequence of chronic vomiting, eating disorders such as bulimia, or gastroesophageal reflux disease. Patients will often report their reflux symptoms; however, some may not. Therefore, oral health providers should obtain a thorough medical history so that they can address this condition. The clinical presentation of erosion due to gastrointestinal reflux is the presence of concave depressions on the palatal and occlusal surfaces of the maxillary teeth and on the buccal and occlusal surfaces of the mandibular teeth (Hattab and Yassin 2000; Litonjua et al. 2003a). The erosive lesions produced as a result of chronic vomiting have been called perimolysis or perimylolysis (Hattab and Yassin 2000). Medication-induced dental erosion has been associated with asthma (Sontag 2000; Sivasithamparam et al. 2002), vitamin C preparations (Eriksson and Angmar-Mansson 1986), and hydrochloric acid for gastric achlorhydria (Hellwig and Lussi 2006; Dugmore and Rock 2003). In general, erosion is a chronic process that patients may or may not be aware of until it has reached an advanced stage. This condition must be detected early if further progression of this condition is to be prevented. A careful medical history, including information about diet, salivary function, and adjunct tooth wear processes as predisposing factors and a lifestyle evaluation are necessary (Fig. 3.4) (Table 3.1).

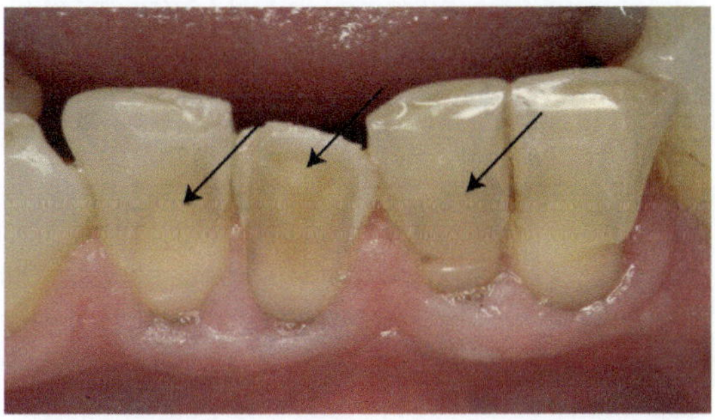

Fig. 3.4 Erosion lesion (*arrows*) due to loss of mineralized dental hard tissue caused by the direct impact of exogenous acids

3.3.1.4 Toothbrushing

3.3.1.4.1 Excessive Toothbrushing

Traumatic toothbrushing is believed to be responsible for the development of gingival lacerations, cementum loss, and root dentin exposure, all of which predispose patients to cervical lesion sensitivity. Mannerberg and associates reported that toothbrushing produces scratches on tooth surfaces that can eventually cease to exist because of the deposition of inorganic substances that precipitate from saliva (Mannerberg 1961). Toothbrushing by itself can eliminate plaque but may not be able to remove stains from tooth surfaces. Alone, toothbrushing may not harm enamel surfaces (Addy 2005). Toothpaste is a potential adjunct oral health-care product that can eliminate stains and superficial deposits because their key ingredient is an abrasive (Addy 2005). Relative dentin abrasivity (RDA) indicates the

Table 3.1 Etiological factors for dental erosion

Extrinsic				Intrinsic
Dietary	Medication	Occupation	Environment/lifestyle	Chronic vomiting
Acidic fruits	Aspirin Asthma medication	Wine tasting	Healthier lifestyle – consuming more fruits/juices	*Bulimia nervosa*
Acidic drinks	Vitamin C	Battery manufacturing Pharmaceutical and biotechnical work	Excessive oral hygiene – tooth brushing habit	*Gastric achlorhydria*
Aerated beverages	Toothpastes Mouthwashes Mouth refresher	Swimmers	Self-inflicting	*Chronic alcoholism*

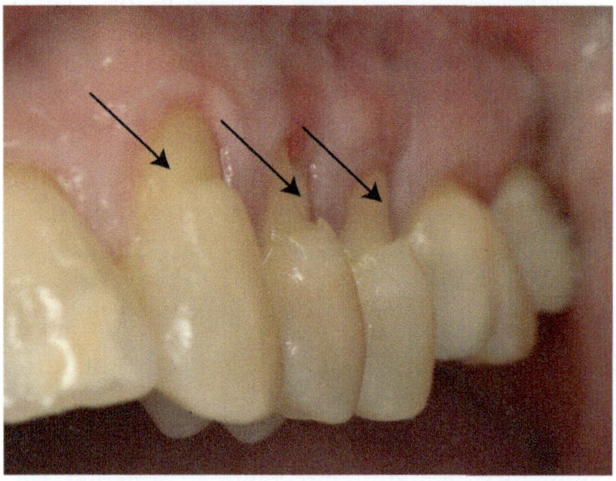

Fig. 3.5 Gingival recession and subsequent abrasion lesion (*arrows*) due to traumatic toothbrushing habit in right-handed patient

degree of abrasivity of toothpastes. Joiner and co-workers performed an in situ study to evaluate toothpastes with various RDAs and found that the amount of enamel wear caused by toothpastes may not be clinically significant (Joiner et al. 2004). However, brushing with toothpaste does abrade dentin, and the rate of wear corresponds to the paste's RDA value (Addy et al. 2002). Absi and colleagues reported that toothbrushing alone could not open the tubule; however, brushing with toothpaste exerted a constructive effect by forming a smear layer and closing the dentinal tubules (Absi et al. 1992). West and associates found that using toothpastes other than silica-based pastes to brush teeth with localized sites of dentin exposure can play a role in the removal of the smear layer, thus opening the tubule and leading to the development of DH (West et al. 2002). Interestingly, some authors have reported that some toothpastes remove the smear layer and then occlude the dentinal tubule with the abrasive particles that they contain (Banfield and Addy 2004; West et al. 2002). Therefore, it can be said that toothbrushing alone or with toothpaste can produce an insignificant change on the enamel surface; however, both types of brushing can enhance tooth wear by the action of a more prevailing process such as erosion (Fig. 3.5).

3.3.1.4.2 Lack of Toothbrushing

Lack of toothbrushing results in the accumulation of plaque. The role of plaque in the etiology of DH is debatable. Published reports indicate that patients who maintain effective plaque control are not affected by DH (Tammaro et al. 2000), whereas those whose root surface is exposed to plaque are predisposed to the development of DH (Trowbridge and Silver 1990; Cox 1994). Kawasaki and colleagues validated the effects of plaque control on dentinal tubule widening and occlusion in association with DH. They created dentin slabs by using human teeth and subjected one group of them to no measures for controlling plaque, a second group to mechanical plaque control with brushing, and a third group to chemical plaque control with chlorhexidine. They found that wider tubules were not associated with plaque control and that occluded tubules were associated with mechanical and chemical plaque-control measures (Kawasaki et al. 2001). Bacteria from dental plaque may penetrate the dentinal tubules and release their products, thereby stimulating the nerve fibers. It has been reported that bacteria can enter the dentinal tubule by dissolving the smear layer and can progress toward the dental pulp, thereby inducing DH (Adriaens et al. 1988). Adriaens and associates found that substantial numbers of viable bacteria are present throughout the radicular dentin of teeth with no periodontal diseases or caries (Adriaens et al. 1988). On the other hand, it is believed that plaque does not contribute to DH, because its incidence is higher among patients with excessive toothbrush abrasion at sites that are almost plaque free (Addy et al. 1987; Addy and Pearce 1994).

3.3.1.5 Abfraction

Abfraction, a new term introduced by Grippo (1991), is associated with cervical lesions that are anticipated to play an important role in the process of tooth wear. It is related to eccentric occlusal loading (Dababneh et al. 1999). The lateral occlusal forces exerted during mastication, parafunction, or malocclusion produce tensile stresses that can result in cusp flexure and may transmit these stresses particularly in the cervical areas, resulting in weakening and eventually cracking in the cervical region around the cementoenamel junction (CEJ) (Lee and Eakle 1984; Hattab and Yassin 2000). The lesion appears to be a V-shaped defect in the cervical areas of the buccal surface

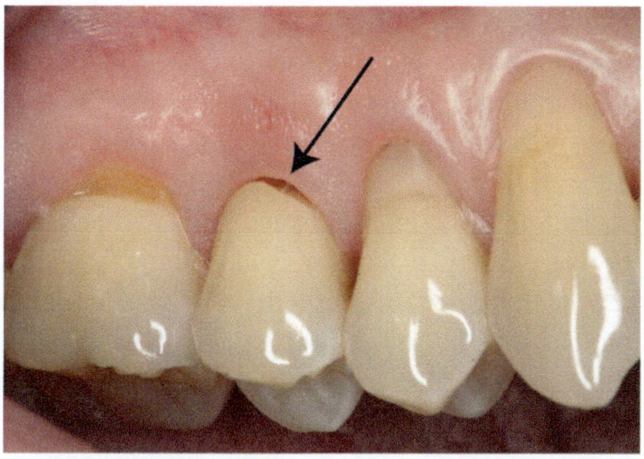

Fig. 3.6 Abfraction-related tooth wear that is related to eccentric occlusal loading

of the teeth; this lesion must be differentiated from tooth abrasion, microfracture (Bevenius et al. 1993), and erosion lesion. Clinical observations have suggested that abfraction lesions are more prevalent in maxillary (upper jaw) incisors (Grippo 1991) and in bruxism patients (Xhonga 1977). Although abfraction can be linked to DH because of the development of cervical cracks and lesions, there is not enough published evidence to suggest that abfraction alone can be a potential etiological factor in tooth wear (Litonjua et al. 2003b). On the other hand, factors such as erosion and abrasion are more potentiating and can occur in combination with abfraction to further elicit the development of DH (Fig. 3.6).

3.3.2 Iatrogenic Factors

Mwangi and colleagues performed a retrospective survey to evaluate the long-term relationship between malocclusion, orthodontic treatment, and tooth wear. They found no significant differences in tooth wear between patients who had or had not received orthodontic treatment. Furthermore, they also reported no correlation between tooth wear and acidic intake in these patients (Mwangi et al. 2009).

Dentin hypersensitivity is also reported after the application of restorative materials, tooth-whitening procedures, and ill-fitting trays with a surplus of tooth-whitening materials (Nathanson 1997). Restorations with a composite material that involves an acid-etching step performed beyond the CEJ margin can also predispose patients to sensitivity. Furthermore, sensitivity can also occur if the dentin tubule that is newly cut during cavity preparation is left exposed during the restorative procedure. The pain associated with restorative sensitivity can occur for a short period of time. However, if the dental pulp tissue is involved because of the process of caries, severe pain that persists for a longer duration must be differentiated from DH. Incorrect use of whitening solutions (bleaching agents) places patients at risk of DH and gingival irritation, particularly when the night guard vital bleaching technique is used (Leonard et al. 1997). Although DH is a common side effect after using bleaching agents, the mechanism of bleaching-associated sensitivity is not fully understood. It has been shown that bleaching agents may change the surface roughness of enamel and predispose teeth to enamel erosion (Azrak et al. 2010). Controlled clinical studies have shown that although some bleaching gels produce some alterations of the enamel surface, these alterations return to normal within 3 months (Turkun et al. 2002). A recent clinical study found that tooth sensitivity is lower (16.7–26.7 %) when hydrogen peroxide bleaching gels are used (Reis et al. 2013). On the other hand, some clinical studies have reported higher levels of tooth sensitivity ranging from 63 % (Marson et al. 2008) to 80 % (Reis et al. 2011). It is recommended that clinical practitioners carefully evaluate exposed dentin, enamel fractures or cracks, large restorations, and cervical erosion because patients with these conditions may be prone to sensitivity after vital tooth bleaching (Nathanson 1997).

3.3.3 Physiological Cause

The CEJ is the anatomical juncture of the enamel that covers the crown and the cementum that covers the root of the teeth. In some patients, enamel and cementum fail to meet at the CEJ, thus resulting in the exposure of some amount of dentin. As the patient ages, the number of teeth with exposed roots increases in association with gingival recession. An increasing number of aged patients with missing natural teeth tend to experience dental extrusion of the opposing tooth, increased gingival recession (Marini et al. 2004), and root exposure, all of which place them at increased risk of DH.

3.3.4 Cementum Loss

Loss of cementum is a multifactorial condition. Exposure of root dentin is apparent in periodontal diseases and is usually associated with gingival recession. It is not uncommon to find exposed root dentin after periodontal surgery, where it can be associated with the healing process. Exposed root dentin is also associated with mechanical trauma such as vigorous toothbrushing.

Gingival recession is a common finding in the periodontal clinic and is characterized by the apical migration of the gingival margin beyond the CEJ. Active periodontal disease (both chronic and acute) may result clinically in gingival recession, bone destruction, and loss of connective tissue attachment. After gingival recession, the root dentin is exposed to the oral cavity, and this exposed root surface is prone to abrasion and erosion. The combination of several predisposing factors makes the exposed dentin tissue very sensitive among patients with periodontal disease. However, it is not uncommon to find gingival recession along with dentin hypersensitivity after some form of periodontal treatment or surgery (Al-Sabbagh et al. 2010). It has been reported that 88 % of people aged 65 years or older have one or more sites of recession. Also, the extent of recession increases with age (Kassab and Cohen 2003). Tammaro and co-workers examined 35 patients with moderate to advanced periodontitis requiring nonsurgical periodontal therapy involving either oral hygiene instruction or scaling and root planning (SRP) and assessed them for the development of root dentin hypersensitivity. They found that the incidence of sensitivity was higher in association with nonsurgical periodontal instrumentation than with oral hygiene instructions with no instrumentation (Tammaro et al. 2000). Canakci and co-workers studied the discomfort levels with respect to pain and DH of 56 patients with chronic periodontitis in response to nonsurgical periodontal treatment and compared them with the discomfort levels of patients after surgical periodontal therapy (osseous, regeneration, gingivectomy, and modified Widman flap). They concluded that the levels of postoperative pain and sensitivity were higher after all surgical periodontal treatments than after nonsurgical therapy and modified Widman flap procedures (Canakci and Canakci 2007). A recent study demonstrated that DH was higher in patients with severe recession. Furthermore, these authors also found an association between DH and good oral hygiene, frequency of toothbrushing, and clinical shape of lesions as V-shaped notches in the cervical areas of canines and first premolars (Fukumoto et al. 2013). It has been suggested that patients with a pronounced scalloped gingival biotype are more prone to gingival recession on the buccal surface of the front teeth than are patients with a flat gingival biotype (Olsson and Lindhe 1991). Overzealous toothbrushing can result in chronic trauma to the gingival margin, resulting in gingival recession and exposure of the root dentin. Furthermore, it has been previously reported that gingival recession is more common among patients with a higher frequency of toothbrushing, especially with a hard toothbrush (Khocht et al. 1993). Gingival recession is a common finding among patients with plaque-free tooth surfaces, probably because of their excessive toothbrushing and excellent oral hygiene practices (Fig. 3.5).

3.3.5 Medical Conditions That Predispose to Dentin Hypersensitivity

The primary medical conditions associated with the risk of dentin hypersensitivity are asthma, bulimia nervosa, gastroesophageal reflux disease, and salivary hypofunction. The prevalence of asthma has increased during the last century. In 2012, 25.7 million adults and 7.0 million children in the USA have asthma, and current estimates suggest that the number of people with asthma increases by approximately 2.9 % every year (Akinbami et al. 2012). Asthma is characterized by the presence of notable air flow obstruction over short periods of time and is reversible with treatment. Asthma treatments are based on the objectives of reducing inflammation by administering anti-inflammatory drugs and releasing blocked airways by administering bronchodilators. Most asthma drugs are administered via inhalers or nebulizers and are inhaled to provide quick relief. Controversy exists among dental practitioners with regard to the effect of these drugs on oral and dental health. Recent studies suggest that patients taking asthma medication are at risk of tooth decay (Boskabady et al. 2012; Reddy et al. 2003), dental erosion (Shaw et al. 2000), and poor periodontal health (McDerra et al. 1998; Ferrazzano et al. 2012b). The factors that predispose asthmatic patients to poor oral health probably result from the pharmacological properties of the medications and altered salivary function and may depend on the composition of the drugs. Ryberg and colleagues reported that, in comparison to nonasthmatic patients, children using β_2 adrenoreceptor agonists to treat asthma exhibited a 26 % decrease in salivary secretion rate, a 70 % increase in the number of streptococcus mutants, a reduction in amylase activity, and an increase in decayed and filled tooth surfaces, thus necessitating special care (Ryberg et al. 1987). Kargul and associates evaluated the pH of interproximal plaque in 30 children aged 6–14 years in relation to medications administered by inhalers and the corresponding effect once saliva had been stimulated by chewing sugar-free gum. They reported that 30 min after the medication was inhaled, the pH of saliva was significantly decreased; however, the pH was higher after the patients chewed gum (Kargul et al. 1998). Altered salivary flow and function can jeopardize the mouth's defensive ability and can subsequently create an environment that can predispose patients to tooth decay. It has been shown that the pH of drugs used to treat asthma (powder and aerosol; pH, 4.76) is lower than the critical pH of enamel (5.5), a finding suggesting that these drugs can dissolve hydroxyapatite (O'Sullivan and Curzon 1998). Although published reports suggest that asthmatic patients are at risk of caries or oral health problems, some studies have shown that there is no association between asthma severity and the potential risk of tooth decay or gingivitis (Bjerkeborn et al. 1987; Eloot et al. 2004). However, some studies have reported that the potential risk of caries among patients who consume oral liquid medications such as syrup is probably due to the high sugar content of these medications (Kenny and Somaya 1989; Reddy et al. 2003).

Recently, case–control studies have suggested a positive association between dental erosion and asthma (Sivasithamparam et al. 2002; Shaw et al. 2000). The prevalence of dental erosion among asthmatic patients taking medications and with an acidic dietary component has been reported to be approximately 35 % (Al-Dlaigan et al. 2002). The etiology of dental erosion in these patients can be attributed to the exposure to both extrinsic acid and intrinsic acid. The source of extrinsic acid can be the acidic dietary intake or acidic medications. On the other hand, the source of intrinsic acid can be the acid present during regurgitation, which is known to be a common symptom among asthmatic patients. In conclusion, asthmatic patients are at risk of oral disease because of the pharmacological action of their medications, altered saliva composition, and exposure to erosive agents, which predispose them to dentin sensitivity.

Published reports indicate that the prevalence of dental erosion is increased among patients with gastroesophageal reflux disease (Barron et al. 2003; Scheutzel 1996), chronic alcoholism (Robb and Smith 1990), and chronic vomiting (Allan 1969). The degree of erosion can be directly linked to the incidence of the disorder and the contact of the acid to the tooth surface, which predisposes it to sensitivity.

Sivasithamparam and colleagues reported that young asthmatic adults display a higher incidence of occlusal erosion than do control subjects, who show more occlusal attrition. Also, despite the evidence of gastroesophageal reflux disease, lingual erosion of the mandibular anterior teeth was not observed, probably because of the protective function of the salivary glands and tongue. The authors suggested that an exogenous source of acid predisposes asthmatic patients to a higher risk of dental erosion (Sivasithamparam et al. 2002). Bulimia nervosa, a disorder characterized by eating exaggerated quantities of food and perpetually self-inducing vomiting, is prevalent among teenage girls and can be associated with fluid and electrolyte imbalance. The degree of erosion can be related to the frequency of vomiting. Valena and associates suggested that erosion due to extrinsic acid can be differentiated from erosion due to intrinsic acid in that the cervical lesions associated with incisal erosion on the lingual surface of mandibular incisors, canines, and premolars are characteristic of bulimia nervosa or gastric esophageal reflux disease (resulting from erosion induced by intrinsic acid) (Valena and Young 2002).

Quality of life is affected by lack of salivary flow, which can lead to difficulties in speaking, eating, tasting, swallowing, and social interaction (Belenguer et al. 2005; Gonzalez et al. 2013). Dry mouth can result from a variety of causes, such as medication, irradiation, salivary gland disease (Sjögren syndrome), and dehydration (Scully 2003). Many drugs can induce hyposalivation, which produces the symptoms of dryness in the mouth. The most common reports of reduced salivary function involve drugs with anticholinergic activity (Wynn and Meiller 2001).

Xerostomia (dry mouth) is a common complication experienced by patients with head and neck cancer. Radiation-induced xerostomia is associated with salivary gland dysfunction; irradiation of the glands can result in extensive tissue damage because of the effects of radiation on cellular DNA. Reports indicate that salivary functions may be reduced within 6–8 months after radiation therapy, and some patients may experience permanent loss of function (Dirix et al. 2006). Wijers et al. surveyed 39 long-term survivors of head and neck cancer treated with radiation therapy; the patients were asked to complete a questionnaire and a visual analog scale (VAS) evaluating the degree of xerostomia they had experienced. Of these patients, 64 % reported moderate to severe long-term xerostomia (Wijers et al. 2002).

The alterations in salivary function experienced by head and neck cancer patients, including salivary hypofunction, lack of protective salivary pellicle formation, and changes in saliva composition, can predispose these patients to long-term oral complications, such as dental caries and mucositis. Treatments such as saliva substitutes, amifostine, pilocarpine (Dirix et al. 2006), and submandibular salivary gland transfer (Jha et al. 2012) have been reported to be efficacious for radiation-induced xerostomia. Jarvinen et al. reported that patients with a low unstimulated rate of saliva flow are five times more likely to experience dental erosion than those with a normal flow rate (Jarvinen et al. 1991).

Sjögren syndrome (SS) is a chronic inflammatory systemic autoimmune disease affecting the exocrine glands, principally the salivary and lacrimal glands. SS is characterized by xerostomia and keratoconjunctivitis sicca (dry eyes), which result from the presence of inflammatory cell infiltrates in the tissues of the exocrine glands (Pedersen and Nauntofte 2001). The disease can also occur in association with autoimmune diseases such as rheumatoid arthritis or systemic lupus erythematosus; in such cases it is referred to as secondary Sjögren syndrome. Xerostomia persisting longer than 3 months is common among patients with SS (Al-Hashimi 2001).

The disruption of normal protective salivary function can result in a wide range of detrimental consequences to the oral cavity. Reduced salivary flow, xerostomia, hyposalivation, and altered salivary composition are some of the main risk factors for tooth decay and demineralization and can also potentiate dentin hypersensitivity, bacterial attack, mucosal irritations, and allergies to various other chemical and microbial insults (Al-Hashimi 2001). Depending on the severity of the disease, the dentist must provide the primary oral care. A multidisciplinary approach should be considered, with the goal of improving patients' quality of life (Gonzalez et al. 2013). Sardenberg et al. reported the case of a 10-year-old boy with SS and suggested that improving quality of life requires early diagnosis and treatment of oral symptoms (Sardenberg et al. 2010). Another case report, by Young et al., describes a patient with tooth wear associated with SS (Young et al. 2001). Clinically, the patient exhibited sialadenosis and xerostomia resulting from SS and signs of extensive loss of enamel on the palatal surfaces of the maxillary anterior teeth, as well as some smooth and dull worn areas accompanied by white and rough surfaces of exposed enamel on maxillary incisors and premolars. Another example of the detrimental effects of reduced salivary flow in SS patients is shown in Fig. 3.7.

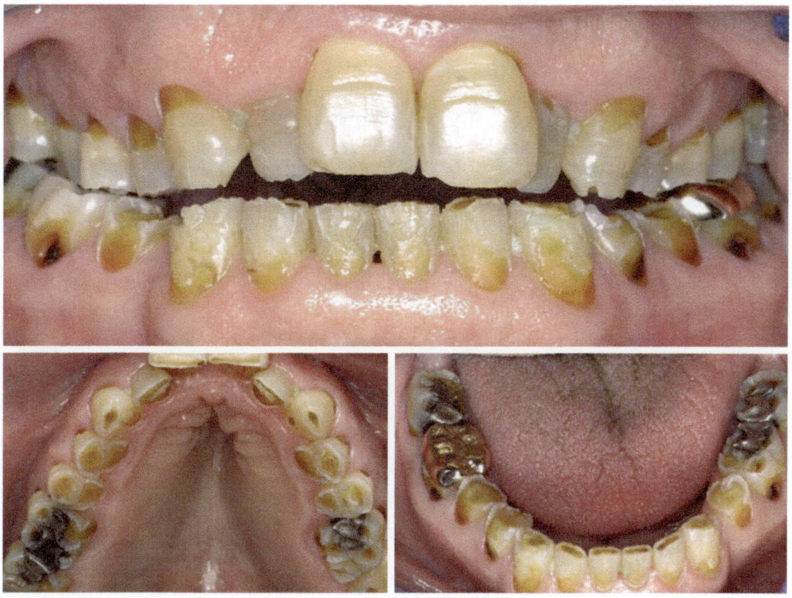

Fig. 3.7 Combined caries-erosion lesions associated with dentin hypersensitivity in a patient suffering from Sjögren syndrome. Soft tissues are shiny due to the lack of saliva

Dehydration is an important cause of salivary dysfunction (Dawes 1987). Lifestyle-linked dehydration (sports related) is a risk factor for xerostomia, which can predispose patients to acid attacks on the tooth surface. These attacks can result in the loss of teeth (Young 2001).

In conclusion, patients with a medical history of eating disorders, asthma, chronic vomiting, dehydration, radiation-induced xerostomia, Sjögren syndrome, chronic alcoholism, or gastro-esophageal disorders may be at a higher risk of oral disease, particularly dental erosion. Dental practitioners, therefore, should pay particular attention to patients with these conditions so that they can provide suitable referrals, encourage good oral health, and deliver effective dental treatment.

References

Absi EG, Addy M, Adams D (1987) Dentine hypersensitivity. A study of the patency of dentinal tubules in sensitive and non-sensitive cervical dentine. J Clin Periodontol 14(5):280–284

Absi EG, Addy M, Adams D (1992) Dentine hypersensitivity–the effect of toothbrushing and dietary compounds on dentine in vitro: an SEM study. J Oral Rehabil 19(2):101–110

Addy M (2005) Tooth brushing, tooth wear and dentine hypersensitivity–are they associated? Int Dent J 55 (4 Suppl 1):261–267

Addy M, Pearce N (1994) Aetiological, predisposing and environmental factors in dentine hypersensitivity. Arch Oral Biol 39(Suppl):33S–38S

Addy M, Mostafa P, Newcombe RG (1987) Dentine hypersensitivity: the distribution of recession, sensitivity and plaque. J Dent 15(6):242–248

Addy M, Hughes J, Pickles MJ, Joiner A, Huntington E (2002) Development of a method in situ to study toothpaste abrasion of dentine. Comparison of 2 products. J Clin Periodontol 29(10):896–900

Adriaens PA, De Boever JA, Loesche WJ (1988) Bacterial invasion in root cementum and radicular dentin of periodontally diseased teeth in humans. A reservoir of periodontopathic bacteria. J Periodontol 59(4): 222–230. doi:10.1902/jop.1988.59.4.222

Akinbami LJ, Moorman JE, Bailey C, Zahran HS, King M, Johnson CA, Liu X (2012) Trends in asthma prevalence, health care use, and mortality in the United States, 2001–2010. NCHS Data Brief 94:1–8

Al-Dlaigan YH, Shaw L, Smith AJ (2002) Is there a relationship between asthma and dental erosion? A case control study. Int J Paediatr Dent 12(3):189–200

Al-Hashimi I (2001) The management of Sjogren's syndrome in dental practice. J Am Dent Assoc (1939) 132(10):1409–1417; quiz 1460–1461

Allan DN (1969) Dental erosion from vomiting. A case report. Br Dent J 126(7):311–312

Al-Sabbagh M, Andreana S, Ciancio SG (2004) Dentinal hypersensitivity: Review of etiology, differential diagnosis, prevalence, and mechanism. J Int Acad Perio 6(1):8–12

Al-Sabbagh M, Beneduce C, Andreana S, Ciancio SG (2010) Incidence and time course of dentinal hypersensitivity after surgical periodontal therapy. Gen Dent 58(1):e14–e19
Arnadottir IB, Holbrook WP, Eggertsson H, Gudmundsdottir H, Jonsson SH, Gudlaugsson JO, Saemundsson SR, Eliasson ST, Agustsdottir H (2010) Prevalence of dental erosion in children: a national survey. Community Dent Oral Epidemiol 38(6): 521–526. doi:10.1111/j.1600-0528.2010.00559.x
Attin T, Buchalla W, Gollner M, Hellwig E (2000) Use of variable remineralization periods to improve the abrasion resistance of previously eroded enamel. Caries Res 34(1):48–52, 16569
Azrak B, Callaway A, Kurth P, Willershausen B (2010) Influence of bleaching agents on surface roughness of sound or eroded dental enamel specimens. J Esthet Restor Dent 22(6):391–399. doi:10.1111/j.1708-8240.2010.00372.x
Banfield N, Addy M (2004) Dentine hypersensitivity: development and evaluation of a model in situ to study tubulepatency. J Clin Periodontol 31(5):325–335. doi:10.1111/j.1600-051X.2004.00488.x
Barron RP, Carmichael RP, Marcon MA, Sandor GK (2003) Dental erosion in gastroesophageal reflux disease. J Can Dent Assoc 69(2):84–89
Bartlett DW, Shah P (2006) A critical review of non-carious cervical (wear) lesions and the role of abfraction, erosion, and abrasion. J Dent Res 85(4): 306–312
Belenguer R, Ramos-Casals M, Brito-Zeron P, del Pino J, Sentis J, Aguilo S, Font J (2005) Influence of clinical and immunological parameters on the health-related quality of life of patients with primary Sjogren's syndrome. Clin Exp Rheumatol 23(3):351–356
Bergstrom J, Lavstedt S (1979) An epidemiologic approach to toothbrushing and dental abrasion. Community Dent Oral Epidemiol 7(1):57–64
Bevenius J, L'Estrange P, Karlsson S, Carlsson GE (1993) Idiopathic cervical lesions: in vivo investigation by oral microendoscopy and scanning electron microscopy. A pilot study. J Oral Rehabil 20(1):1–9
Bhatti SA, Walsh TF, Douglas CW (1994) Ethanol and pH levels of proprietary mouthrinses. Community Dent Health 11(2):71–74
Bishop K, Kelleher M, Briggs P, Joshi R (1997) Wear now? An update on the etiology of tooth wear. Quintessence Int (Berlin, Germany: 1985) 28(5): 305–313
Bjerkeborn K, Dahllof G, Hedlin G, Lindell M, Modeer T (1987) Effect of disease severity and pharmacotherapy of asthma on oral health in asthmatic children. Scand J Dent Res 95(2):159–164
Boskabady M, Nematollahi H, Boskabady MH (2012) Effect of inhaled medication and inhalation technique on dental caries in asthmatic patients. Iranian Red Crescent Med J 14(12):816–821. doi:10.5812/ircmj.4658
Brannstrom M (1965) The surface of sensitive dentine. An experimental study using replication. Odontol Revy 16(4):293–299
Brannstrom M (1986) The hydrodynamic theory of dentinal pain: sensation in preparations, caries, and the dentinal crack syndrome. J Endod 12(10):453–457. doi:10.1016/s0099-2399(86)80198-4
Brannstrom M, Garberoglio R (1980) Occlusion of dentinal tubules under superficial attrited dentine. Swed Dent J 4(3):87–91
Canakci CF, Canakci V (2007) Pain experienced by patients undergoing different periodontal therapies. J Am Dent Assoc (1939) 138(12):1563–1573
Centerwall BS, Armstrong CW, Funkhouser LS, Elzay RP (1986) Erosion of dental enamel among competitive swimmers at a gas-chlorinated swimming pool. Am J Epidemiol 123(4):641–647
Cox CF (1994) Etiology and treatment of root hypersensitivity. Am J Dent 7(5):266–270
Cunha-Cruz J, Wataha JC, Heaton LJ, Rothen M, Sobieraj M, Scott J, Berg J (2013) The prevalence of dentin hypersensitivity in general dental practices in the northwest United States. J Am Dent Assoc (1939) 144(3):288–296
Curro FA (1990) Tooth hypersensitivity in the spectrum of pain. Dent Clin N Am 34(3):429–437
Dababneh RH, Khouri AT, Addy M (1999) Dentine hypersensitivity – an enigma? A review of terminology, mechanisms, aetiology and management. Br Dent J 187(11):606–611. doi:10.1038/sj.bdj.4800345a; discussion 603
Davis WB, Winter PJ (1980) The effect of abrasion on enamel and dentine and exposure to dietary acid. Br Dent J 148(11–12):253–256
Dawes C (1987) Physiological factors affecting salivary flow rate, oral sugar clearance, and the sensation of dry mouth in man. J Dent Res 66(Spec No):648–653
Dirix P, Nuyts S, Van den Bogaert W (2006) Radiation-induced xerostomia in patients with head and neck cancer: a literature review. Cancer 107(11): 2525–2534. doi:10.1002/cncr.22302
Dugmore CR, Rock WP (2003) Asthma and tooth erosion. Is there an association? Int J Paediatr Dent 13(6): 417–424
Dyer D, Addy M, Newcombe RG (2000) Studies in vitro of abrasion by different manual toothbrush heads and a standard toothpaste. J Clin Periodontol 27(2): 99–103
Ehlen LA, Marshall TA, Qian F, Wefel JS, Warren JJ (2008) Acidic beverages increase the risk of in vitro tooth erosion. Nutr Res 28(5):299–303. doi:10.1016/j.nutres.2008.03.001
Eloot AK, Vanobbergen JN, De Baets F, Martens LC (2004) Oral health and habits in children with asthma related to severity and duration of condition. Eur J Paediatr Dent 5(4):210–215
Eriksson JH, Angmar-Mansson B (1986) Erosion due to vitamin C tablets. Tandlakartidningen 78(10): 541–544
Ferrazzano GF, Coda M, Cantile T, Sangianantoni G, Ingenito A (2012a) SEM investigation on casein phosphopeptides capability in contrasting cola drinks enamel erosion: an in vitro preliminary study. Eur J Paediatr Dent 13(4):285–288

Ferrazzano GF, Sangianantoni G, Cantile T, Amato I, Ingenito A, Noschese P (2012b) Dental health in asthmatic children: a South Italy study. J Dent Child (Chic) 79(3):170–175

Fukumoto Y, Horibe M, Inagaki Y, Oishi K, Tamaki N, Ito HO, Nagata T (2013) Association of gingival recession and other factors with the presence of dentin hypersensitivity. Odontology. doi:10.1007/s10266-012-0099-5

Glaros AG (1981) Incidence of diurnal and nocturnal bruxism. J Prosthet Dent 45(5):545–549

Gonzalez S, Sung H, Sepulveda D, Gonzalez M, Molina C (2013) Oral manifestations and their treatment in Sjogren's syndrome. Oral Dis. doi:10.1111/odi.12105

Gray A, Ferguson MM, Wall JG (1998) Wine tasting and dental erosion. Case report. Aust Dent J 43(1): 32–34

Grenby TH, Phillips A, Desai T, Mistry M (1989) Laboratory studies of the dental properties of soft drinks. Br J Nutr 62(2):451–464

Grippo JO (1991) Abfractions: a new classification of hard tissue lesions of teeth. J Esthet Dent 3(1): 14–19

Grippo JO, Simring M, Schreiner S (2004) Attrition, abrasion, corrosion and abfraction revisited: a new perspective on tooth surface lesions. J Am Dent Assoc (1939) 135(8):1109–1118; quiz 1163–1165

Hattab FN, Yassin OM (2000) Etiology and diagnosis of tooth wear: a literature review and presentation of selected cases. Int J Prosthodont 13(2):101–107

Hellwig E, Lussi A (2006) Oral hygiene products and acidic medicines. Monogr Oral Sci 20:112–118. doi:10.1159/000093358

Jaeggi T, Lussi A (1999) Toothbrush abrasion of erosively altered enamel after intraoral exposure to saliva: an in situ study. Caries Res 33(6):455–461, 16551

Jarvinen VK, Rytomaa II, Heinonen OP (1991) Risk factors in dental erosion. J Dent Res 70(6):942–947

Jha N, Harris J, Seikaly H, Jacobs JR, McEwan AJ, Robbins KT, Grecula J, Sharma AK, Ang KK (2012) A phase II study of submandibular gland transfer prior to radiation for prevention of radiation-induced xerostomia in head-and-neck cancer (RTOG 0244). Int J Radiat Oncol Biol Phys 84(2):437–442. doi:10.1016/j.ijrobp.2012.02.034

Johansson AK, Lingstrom P, Imfeld T, Birkhed D (2004) Influence of drinking method on tooth-surface pH in relation to dental erosion. Eur J Oral Sci 112(6): 484–489. doi:10.1111/j.1600-0722.2004.00172.x

Johnson GK, Sivers JE (1987) Attrition, abrasion and erosion: diagnosis and therapy. Clin Prev Dent 9(5):12–16

Johnson RH, Zulqar-Nain BJ, Koval JJ (1982) The effectiveness of an electro-ionizing toothbrush in the control of dentinal hypersensitivity. J Periodontol 53(6):353–359. doi:10.1902/jop.1982.53.6.353

Joiner A, Pickles MJ, Tanner C, Weader E, Doyle P (2004) An in situ model to study the toothpaste abrasion of enamel. J Clin Periodontol 31(6):434–438. doi:10.1111/j.1600-051X.2004.00497.x

Kaidonis JA (2008) Tooth wear: the view of the anthropologist. Clin Oral Investig 12(Suppl 1):S21–S26. doi:10.1007/s00784-007-0154-8

Kargul B, Tanboga I, Ergeneli S, Karakoc F, Dagli E (1998) Inhaler medicament effects on saliva and plaque pH in asthmatic children. J Clin Pediatr Dent 22(2):137–140

Kassab MM, Cohen RE (2003) The etiology and prevalence of gingival recession. J Am Dent Assoc (1939) 134(2):220–225

Kawasaki A, Ishikawa K, Suge T, Shimizu H, Suzuki K, Matsuo T, Ebisu S (2001) Effects of plaque control on the patency and occlusion of dentine tubules in situ. J Oral Rehabil 28(5):439–449, jor682 [pii]

Kenny DJ, Somaya P (1989) Sugar load of oral liquid medications on chronically ill children. J Can Dent Assoc 55(1):43–46

Khocht A, Simon G, Person P, Denepitiya JL (1993) Gingival recession in relation to history of hard toothbrush use. J Periodontol 64(9):900–905. doi:10.1902/jop.1993.64.9.900

Kitchin PC (1941) Cervical exposure and abrasion in human teeth for different age classes. Science 94(2429):65–66. doi:10.1126/science.94.2429.65

Knight T (1969) Erosion-abrasion. J Dent Assoc S Afr 24(10):310–316

Lee WC, Eakle WS (1984) Possible role of tensile stress in the etiology of cervical erosive lesions of teeth. J Prosthet Dent 52(3):374–380

Leonard RH, Jr., Haywood VB, Phillips C (1997) Risk factors for developing tooth sensitivity and gingival irritation associated with nightguard vital bleaching. Quintessence Int (Berlin, Germany: 1985) 28(8): 527–534

Levitch LC, Bader JD, Shugars DA, Heymann HO (1994) Non-carious cervical lesions. J Dent 22(4):195–207

Li H, Zou Y, Ding G (2012) Dietary factors associated with dental erosion: a meta-analysis. PloS one 7(8):e42626. doi:10.1371/journal.pone.0042626

Litonjua LA, Andreana S, Bush PJ, Cohen RE (2003a) Tooth wear: attrition, erosion, and abrasion. Quintessence Int (Berlin, Germany: 1985) 34(6): 435–446

Litonjua LA, Andreana S, Bush PJ, Tobias TS, Cohen RE (2003b) Noncarious cervical lesions and abfractions: a re-evaluation. J Am Dent Assoc (1939) 134(7): 845–850

Litonjua LA, Andreana S, Bush PJ, Tobias TS, Cohen RE (2004) Wedged cervical lesions produced by toothbrushing. Am J Dent 17(4):237–240

Mannerberg F (1961) Changes in the enamel surface in cases of erosion. A replica study. Arch Oral Biol 4:59–62

Marini MG, Greghi SL, Passanezi E, Sant'ana AC (2004) Gingival recession: prevalence, extension and severity in adults. J Appl Oral Sci 12(3):250–255

Marson FC, Sensi LG, Vieira LC, Araujo E (2008) Clinical evaluation of in-office dental bleaching treatments with and without the use of light-activation sources. Oper Dent 33(1):15–22. doi:10.2341/07-57

McDerra EJ, Pollard MA, Curzon ME (1998) The dental status of asthmatic British school children. Pediatr Dent 20(4):281–287

Meurman JH, ten Cate JM (1996) Pathogenesis and modifying factors of dental erosion. Eur J Oral Sci 104(2(Pt 2)):199–206

Murphy TR (1964) The relationship between attritional facets and the occlusal plane in aboriginal australians. Arch Oral Biol 9:269–280

Mwangi CW, Richmond S, Hunter ML (2009) Relationship between malocclusion, orthodontic treatment, and tooth wear. Am J Orthod Dentofacial Orthop 136(4):529–535. doi:10.1016/j.ajodo.2007.11.030

Nathanson D (1997) Vital tooth bleaching: sensitivity and pulpal considerations. J Am Dent Assoc (1939) 128(Suppl):41S–44S

Nekrashevych Y, Stosser L (2003) Protective influence of experimentally formed salivary pellicle on enamel erosion. An in vitro study. Caries Res 37(3):225–231, 70449

O'Sullivan EA, Curzon MEJ (1998) Drug treatments for asthma may cause erosive tooth damage. BMJ 317(7161):820

Olsson M, Lindhe J (1991) Periodontal characteristics in individuals with varying form of the upper central incisors. J Clin Periodontol 18(1):78–82

Osborne-Smith KL, Burke FJ, Wilson NH (1999) The aetiology of the non-carious cervical lesion. Int Dent J 49(3):139–143

Padbury AD, Ash MM Jr (1974) Abrasion caused by three methods of toothbrushing. J Periodontol 45(6): 434–438. doi:10.1902/jop.1974.45.6.434

Pedersen AM, Nauntofte B (2001) Primary Sjogren's syndrome: oral aspects on pathogenesis, diagnostic criteria, clinical features and approaches for therapy. Expert Opin Pharmacother 2(9):1415–1436. doi:10.1517/14656566.2.9.1415

Petersen PE, Gormsen C (1991) Oral conditions among German battery factory workers. Community Dent Oral Epidemiol 19(2):104–106

Phaneuf EA, Harrington JH, Dale PP, Shklar G (1962) Automatic toothbrush: a new reciprocating action. J Am Dent Assoc (1939) 65:12–25

Piangprach T, Hengtrakool C, Kukiattrakoon B, Kedjarune-Leggat U (2009) The effect of salivary factors on dental erosion in various age groups and tooth surfaces. J Am Dent Assoc (1939) 140(9):1137–1143

Radentz WH, Barnes GP, Cutright DE (1976) A survey of factors possibly associated with cervical abrasion of tooth surfaces. J Periodontol 47(3):148–154. doi:10.1902/jop.1976.47.3.148

Reddy DK, Hegde AM, Munshi AK (2003) Dental caries status of children with bronchial asthma. J Clin Pediatr Dent 27(3):293–295

Reis A, Dalanhol AP, Cunha TS, Kossatz S, Loguercio AD (2011) Assessment of tooth sensitivity using a desensitizer before light-activated bleaching. Oper Dent 36(1):12–17. doi:10.2341/10-148-cr

Reis A, Kossatz S, Martins G, Loguercio A (2013) Efficacy of and effect on tooth sensitivity of in-office bleaching gel concentrations: a randomized clinical trial. Oper Dent. doi:10.2341/12-140-c

Rimondini L, Baroni C, Carrassi A (1995) Ultrastructure of hypersensitive and non-sensitive dentine. A study on replica models. J Clin Periodontol 22(12):899–902

Rirattanapong P, Vongsavan K, Suratit R, Tanaiutchawoot N, Charoenchokdilok V, Jeansuwannagorn S, Yoddee M (2012) Effect of various forms of calcium in dental products on human enamel microhardness in vitro. Southeast Asian J Trop Med Public Health 43(4):1053–1058

Robb ND, Smith BG (1990) Prevalence of pathological tooth wear in patients with chronic alcoholism. Br Dent J 169(11):367–369

Ryberg M, Moller C, Ericson T (1987) Effect of beta 2-adrenoceptor agonists on saliva proteins and dental caries in asthmatic children. J Dent Res 66(8):1404–1406

Sangnes G, Gjermo P (1976) Prevalence of oral soft and hard tissue lesions related to mechanical toothcleansing procedures. Community Dent Oral Epidemiol 4(2):77–83

Sardenberg F, Goursand D, Polletto LT, Vale MP, Zarzar PM, Paiva SM (2010) Oral manifestations and treatment of a child with Sjogren's syndrome. J Dent Child (Chic) 77(2):102–105

Scheutzel P (1996) Etiology of dental erosion–intrinsic factors. Eur J Oral Sci 104(2(Pt 2)):178–190

Scully C (2003) Drug effects on salivary glands: dry mouth. Oral Dis 9(4):165–176

Shaw L, al-Dlaigan YH, Smith A (2000) Childhood asthma and dental erosion. ASDC J Dent Child 67(2):102–106, 182

Sivasithamparam K, Young WG, Jirattanasopa V, Priest J, Khan F, Harbrow D, Daley TJ (2002) Dental erosion in asthma: a case–control study from south east Queensland. Aust Dent J 47(4):298–303

Smith BG, Knight JK (1984) A comparison of patterns of tooth wear with aetiological factors. Br Dent J 157(1):16–19

Sontag SJ (2000) Gastroesophageal reflux disease and asthma. J Clin Gastroenterol 30(3 Suppl):S9–S30

Tammaro S, Wennstrom JL, Bergenholtz G (2000) Root-dentin sensitivity following non-surgical periodontal treatment. J Clin Periodontol 27(9):690–697

Trowbridge HO, Silver DR (1990) A review of current approaches to in-office management of tooth hypersensitivity. Dent Clin N Am 34(3):561–581

Turkun M, Sevgican F, Pehlivan Y, Aktener BO (2002) Effects of 10% carbamide peroxide on the enamel surface morphology: a scanning electron microscopy study. J Esthet Restor Dent 14(4):238–244

Valena V, Young WG (2002) Dental erosion patterns from intrinsic acid regurgitation and vomiting. Aust Dent J 47(2):106–115

West NX, Hughes JA, Addy M (2002) Dentine hypersensitivity: the effects of brushing toothpaste on etched and unetched dentine in vitro. J Oral Rehabil 29(2):167–174, 851 [pii]

Westergaard J, Larsen IB, Holmen L, Larsen AI, Jorgensen B, Holmstrup P, Suadicani P, Gyntelberg F (2001) Occupational exposure to airborne proteolytic enzymes and lifestyle risk factors for dental erosion–a cross-sectional study. Occup Med (Oxford, England) 51(3):189–197

Wijers OB, Levendag PC, Braaksma MM, Boonzaaijer M, Visch LL, Schmitz PI (2002) Patients with head and neck cancer cured by radiation therapy: a survey of the dry mouth syndrome in long-term survivors. Head Neck 24(8):737–747. doi:10.1002/hed.10129

Wynn RL, Meiller TF (2001) Drugs and dry mouth. Gen Dent 49(1):10–12, 14

Xhonga FA (1977) Bruxism and its effect on the teeth. J Oral Rehabil 4(1):65–76

Yoshiyama M, Noiri Y, Ozaki K, Uchida A, Ishikawa Y, Ishida H (1990) Transmission electron microscopic characterization of hypersensitive human radicular dentin. J Dent Res 69(6):1293–1297

Young WG (2001) The oral medicine of tooth wear. Aust Dent J 46(4):236–250; quiz 306

Young W, Khan F, Brandt R, Savage N, Razek AA, Huang Q (2001) Syndromes with salivary dysfunction predispose to tooth wear: case reports of congenital dysfunction of major salivary glands, Prader-Willi, congenital rubella, and Sjogren's syndromes. Oral Surg Oral Med Oral Pathol Oral Radiol Endod 92(1):38–48. doi:10.1067/moe.2001.113549

Zandim DL, Correa FO, Rossa Junior C, Sampaio JE (2008) In vitro evaluation of the effect of natural orange juices on dentin morphology. Braz Oral Res 22(2):176–183, S1806-83242008000200014 [pii]

Zero DT (1996) Etiology of dental erosion–extrinsic factors. Eur J Oral Sci 104(2 (Pt 2)):162–177

Zero DT, Lussi A (2005) Erosion–chemical and biological factors of importance to the dental practitioner. Int Dent J 55(4 Suppl 1):285–290

Zimmer S, Ozturk M, Barthel CR, Bizhang M, Jordan RA (2011) Cleaning efficacy and soft tissue trauma after use of manual toothbrushes with different bristle stiffness. J Periodontol 82(2):267–271. doi:10.1902/jop.2010.100328

4 Diagnosis of Dentin Hypersensitivity

Cornelius Tokunbo Bamise

Abstract

Diagnosis of dentin hypersensitivity involves holistic assessment of the sufferer, particularly the condition of the involved tooth and to identify the cause of the pain or discomfort in order to prescribe appropriate treatment. Knowledge of the physiology of pain and methods of interpreting it with available clinical diagnostic devices is essential to reach a proper diagnosis. The history of the patient's pain is the first clinical data the dentist must collect and consider with careful attention being paid to its characteristics as revealed by the patient's responses, such as the type, duration, frequency, stimulating factors, and disturbed oral functions. Associating patient's features and other factors capable of exposing dentin and opening up the tubules must be well explored. Ultimately, correct diagnosis necessitates awareness of clinical conditions which are similar in their presenting features. Diverse standardized stimuli and means of quantifying the pain of dentin hypersensitivity are discussed in this chapter.

4.1 Introduction

Diagnosis is the art of identifying a problem; in this instance, a condition or disease entity and using scientific knowledge to determine its causative factors. Diagnosis commences with history and a thorough clinical and radiographic examination of the patient particularly of the tissue in question. It includes the patient's social situation and sometimes culture. With respect to dentin hypersensitivity, it is identified by pain (sensitivity) which is triggered by a stimulus to the exposed dentin – the particularity being that this pain is similar to that of other dental disorders of different etiology and, therefore, requiring a different treatment modality. Hence, the need for proper case evaluation and correct diagnosis (Fig. 4.1).

Holland and coworkers (1997) described dentin hypersensitivity as a condition that manifests as a brief and acute pain that cannot be attributed to any other form of dental pathology or defect. Dentin hypersensitivity is a painful clinical condition which requires knowledge of the neuroanatomy of the pulp dentin complex, the physiology of pain and methods of interpreting it to reach a correct diagnosis.

C.T. Bamise
Department of Restorative Dentistry,
Faculty of Dentistry, College of Health Sciences,
Obafemi Awolowo University, Ile-Ife,
Osun-State, Nigeria
e-mail: bamisect@yahoo.com

S. Taha, B.H. Clarkson (eds.), *Clinician's Guide to the Diagnosis and Management of Tooth Sensitivity*,
DOI 10.1007/978-3-642-45164-5_4, © Springer-Verlag Berlin Heidelberg 2014

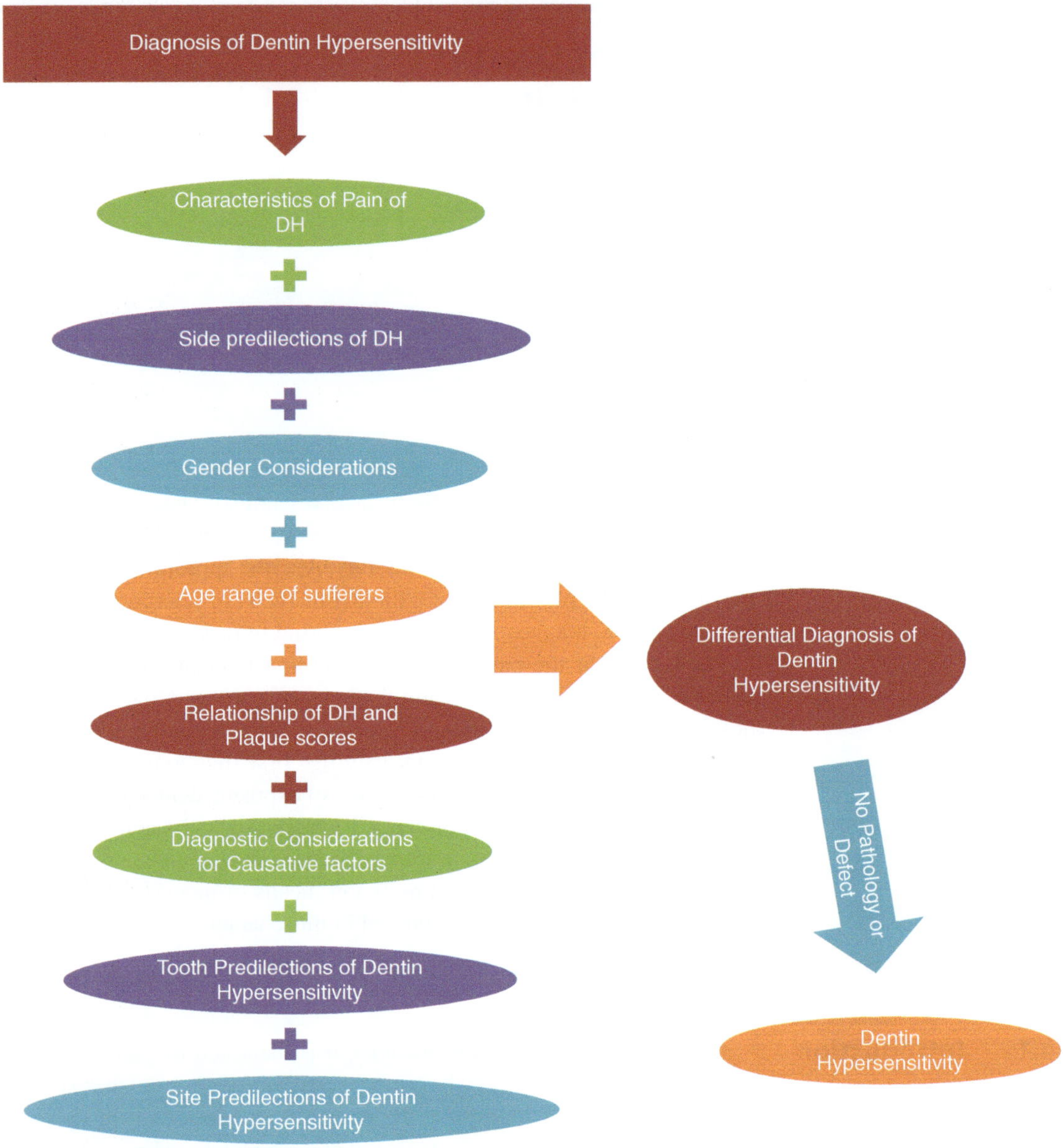

Fig. 4.1 Basic steps in the diagnosis of dentin hypersensitivity

4.2 Innervation of Human Dentin

The dental pulp is a highly innervated organ (Trowbridge 1985; Ten Cate 1994). Nerves enter the pulp through the apical foramen with afferent blood vessels and form neurovascular bundles. They traverse the root canal until they reach the pulp chamber, where the nerve fibers commence to divide and send branches to the surrounding coronal dentin. The nerves form an interlacing network as they approach the subodontoblastic region, known as the subodontoblastic plexus of Raschkow. Here, the myelinated fibers lose their myelin and become free nerve endings. It is estimated that as each nerve fiber enters the pulp, it branches into eight terminal fibers at the pulp-dentin interface. Gunji (1982) classified the nerve endings of these branches into four types: (1)

Marginal fibers, found throughout the peripheral pulp, constitute most of the nerve endings and usually do not reach the predentin. (2) Simple predentinal fibers which reach as far as the predentin. (3) Complex predentinal fibers which arborize profusely within the predentin. (4) Dentinal fibers, the rarest of all, are nerves that pass through the predentin and enter the dentinal tubules, without any branching.

It is estimated that the percentage of dentinal tubules which contain nerve fibrils is 25 % in the pulp horns, 15 % in the coronal dentin, and 10 % in the radicular dentin (Holland 1981). Also, the nerve fibrils may extend up to 1 mm into the dentinal tubule (Lilja 1980). The nerve bundles that enter the tooth are known to consist of sensory afferent nerves, which arise from the trigeminal (5th cranial) nerve, as well as sympathetic branches that arise from the superior cervical ganglion. Some of these nerve fibers are myelinated and others are nonmyelinated. The sympathetic nerve fibers are known to modulate the microcirculation of the dental pulp by controlling the contractions of the smooth muscle cells of the arterioles and the precapillaries.

The sensory nerves in contrast are of two types: A (myelinated) and C (nonmyelinated) nerve fibers. The majority of A fibers are of the A-delta type, which has a diameter range from 1 to 4 μm; they conduct impulses in 4–30 m/s. About 1 % of the A fibers are of the A-beta type, which has a diameter of 6–12 μm and conducts impulses in a faster rate as high as 48 m/s (Narhi et al. 1982a). The unmyelinated C-type nerve fibers have a diameter range of 0.4–1.2 μm and conduct impulses at a rate of 0.5–2 m/s.

4.2.1 Clinical Implications for Intrapulpal Sensory Nerve Fibers

The A-delta fibers have a small diameter and therefore a slower conduction velocity than other types of A fibers, but their conduction velocity is faster than C fibers. The A fibers transmit pain directly to the thalamus, generating a fast, sharp pain that is easily localized. The C fibers are influenced by many modulating interneurons before reaching the thalamus, resulting in a slow pain, which is characterized as dull and aching. The A fibers respond to various stimuli such as probing, drilling, and hypertonic solutions through the hydrodynamic effect (Braennstroem and Astroem 1964; Andrew and Matthews 2000; Narhi 1985; Narhi et al. 1992a).

This effect depends on the movement of the dentinal fluid in the dentinal tubules in response to a stimulus. Although the normally slow capillary outward movement does not stimulate the nerve endings and cause pain (Matthews and Vongsavan 1994; Pashley 1990; Vongsavan and Matthews 2007), rapid fluid flow, as in the case of desiccating or drying dentin, is more intense and is likely to activate the pulpal nociceptors (Braennstroem and Astroem 1964).

Thermal stimuli cause fluid movement through the dentinal tubules, resulting in a painful sensation in a tooth with a viable sensory pulp (Trowbridge 1985, 2003). This response is due to the rapid temperature change that causes a sudden fluid flow within the tubules and deforms the cell membranes of the free nerve endings exciting the A-delta fibers. A gradual change in temperature, however, does not cause an immediate pain response because this elicits a response from the C fibers (Bender 2000; Trowbridge et al. 1980; Narhi et al. 1982b).

Application of cold decreases the blood flow because of its vasoconstrictive effect on the blood vessels. If this application is continued, anoxia results and the A fibers cease to function. With continuous application of heat, the C fibers are affected: vasodilation temporarily increases intrapulpal pressure and causes intense pain (Bender 2000).

Hypertonic solutions activate the intradental nerves through osmotic pressure (Narhi et al. 1992a; Vongsavan and Matthews 2007; Pashley 1986; Anderson et al. 1967), manifested clinically by the pain that results when saturated sucrose solutions come into constant contact with sensitive dentin. This sensitivity is a direct response to the stimulation of the A fibers. Another example is the use of an etchant on the dentinal surface. The osmotic pressure of the acid used for etching the dentin is as important as the acid's chemical composition in the induction of pain because this osmotic pressure causes the outward fluid flow in the tubules, together with aspiration of the odontoblastic nucleus (Anderson et al. 1967; Narhi et al. 1992b; Narhi and Hirvonen 1987).

The ionic concentration of the material also affects the reduction of pain in the sensitive dentin. A normally irritant substance such as potassium chloride temporarily relieves pain because the high concentration of potassium temporarily blocks the conduction of nerve impulses, causing a hyperpolarization that decreases the excitability of the nerve fibers. This hyperpolarization is the basis for the addition of potassium ions to dentifrices to control dentin hypersensitivity.

4.3 Characteristics of Pain of Dentin Hypersensitivity and Associated Factors

Dentin hypersensitivity can be viewed as a symptom complex rather than a true disease. Clinically, it is not associated with obvious tissue damage, but the symptoms indicate potential damage, with constant erosion and attrition of enamel or cementum and a concomitant pulpal response (Curro 1990). The chief symptom of dentin hypersensitivity is pain characterized by rapid onset, sharpness, and short duration. Occasionally, it may persist for a variable time as a dull or vague sensation in the affected tooth after removal of the stimulus. Tactile (toothbrushing and digital probing), thermal (hot and cold), and chemical (acids and sweets) stimuli, as well as exposure to air, can elicit painful responses from individuals with hypersensitive teeth. Brannstrom and Astrom (1972) believed that pain from heat takes longer to develop than pain from cold because heat causes inward movement of the tubular fluid, while the outward movement caused by cold is more rapidly developing (Drisko 2002). Although at times pulpal inflammation complicates the symptomatology, dentin hypersensitivity differs from pain arising in the pulp due to inflammation. Patients can readily locate the source of discomfort or pain when a stimulus is applied to a hypersensitive tooth.

A patient that suffers from dentin hypersensitivity may perceive an exaggerated, intense pain or a more continuous pain stimulus of longer duration which would not be expected to originate only from a hydrodynamic stimulus. The latter is likely to be associated with pulp inflammation. This is because A fibers are relatively insensitive to inflammatory mediators, whereas C fibers may take active part in the development of pulpal inflammation (Olgart and Kerezoudis 1994). Stimuli such as heat, cold, osmotic change, and acid can start an episode of pulpal pain that may last several minutes to many hours and it is usually difficult to locate. Chewing can also be a source of stimulus for pulpal pain, due to hydraulic action, osmotic effects, or trauma.

Dentin hypersensitivity is usually a chronic condition with acute episodes; the dentin that is freshly cut or has recently been curetted will respond to the same cold, heat, osmotic, and acid stimuli in an acute manner. Following cavity preparation, or curettage, the dentin may "heal" due to mineral formation which blocks the tubules, but if "healing" does not occur, the tooth may respond chronically to stimuli that are usually not considered as noxious (Curro 1990).

The history of the patient's pain is the first clinical data that the dentist must collect and consider. The dentist should pay careful attention to the patient's answers about the pain, such as the type, duration, frequency, aggravating factors, effect of analgesics, and tenderness when biting. The nature of the pain described by most patients seeking treatment for dentin hypersensitivity is a sharp pain of short duration (Orchardson and Collins 1987a; Andrej 2002; Canadian Advisory Board on Dentin Hypersensitivity 2003).

The frequency of each episode of pain of dentin hypersensitivity is variable and dependent, somewhat, on the initiating stimulus and is patient dependent. Cold or heat has been described as the most potent stimuli (Canadian Advisory Board on Dentin Hypersensitivity 2003; Orchardson and Collins 1987b; Irwin and McCusker 1997; Rees 2000). The episodic pain associated with dentin hypersensitivity may last from months to years as reported by Schuurs et al. (1995). Taani and Awartani (2002) in a hospital-based study population of 302 subjects reported that 14–23 % claimed their sensitivity had lasted from 1 to 5 years.

Drinking cold water was one function that was severely interfered with in a study by Bamise et al. (2007) with slightly lower percentages of the volunteers mentioning brushing and eating. Taani and Awartani (2002) reported that about 64 % of their patients with dentin hypersensitivity reported that it did not interfere with eating and toothbrushing. The hypersensitivity reported when drinking cold water was explained by the fact that drinking water gains access to more sites in the mouth.

4.3.1 Gender Considerations in the Diagnosis of Dentin Hypersensitivity

Please refer to Sect. 1.3.

4.3.2 Age Range of Sufferers of Dentin Hypersensitivity

Please refer to Sect. 1.3.

4.3.3 Side and Site Predilections of Dentin Hypersensitivity

Please refer to Sect. 1.3.

4.3.4 Tooth Predilection for Dentin Hypersensitivity

Please refer to Sect. 1.3.

4.3.5 Relationship of Dentin Hypersensitivity and Plaque Scores

Please refer to Sect. Lack of Toothbrushing in Chap. 3.

4.4 Diagnostic Considerations for Causative Factors of Dentin Hypersensitivity

Management of a patient suffering from dentin hypersensitivity should be based on a correct diagnosis of the condition by the dentist, who should be aware of other clinical conditions (Sect. 4.3) which are similar in their presenting features (Dababneh et al. 1999). Conditions that lead to enamel loss and exposure of dentin should be carefully evaluated and diagnosed. As discussed earlier, in Sect. 3.3.1, these conditions place the teeth at a higher risk for DH.

Tooth surface loss caused by abfraction, abrasion, or erosion is assumed to progress slowly, a cumulative lifetime process, which is extremely difficult to diagnose in early stages. Sometimes, no obvious changes can be observed on the teeth for many years.

4.5 Differential Diagnosis of Dentin Hypersensitivity

The pain associated with hypersensitive teeth arises when the dentin is exposed and typically occurs in response to chemical, thermal, tactile, or osmotic stimuli. In patients with suspected dentin hypersensitivity due to positive findings in the screening and history, thorough differential diagnosis is very important to eliminate all other forms of orofacial pain.

Several conditions may elicit the same clinical symptoms as dentin hypersensitivity. These include:

- Cracked tooth syndrome
- Fractured restorations
- Chipped teeth
- Caries
- Post-restorative sensitivity
- Palatal-gingival groove
- Hypoplastic enamel
- Improperly insulated metallic restorations
- Teeth in acute hyperfunction

A careful differential diagnosis, therefore, is required to rule out alternative causes of pain. This should include, as mentioned earlier, a

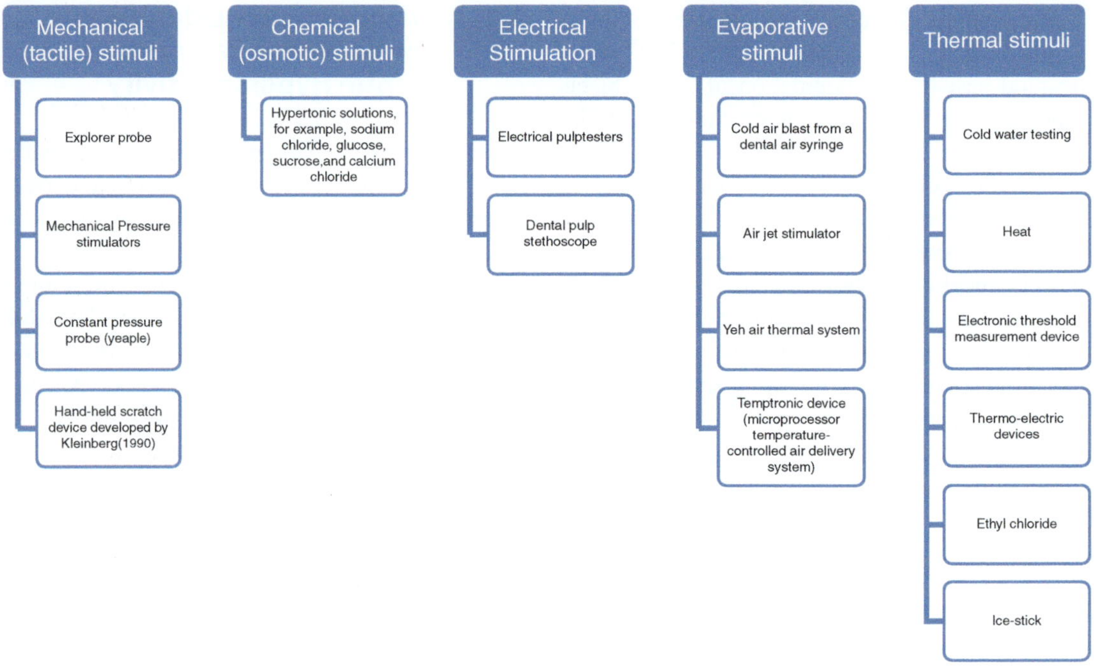

Fig. 4.2 Stimuli to assess dentin hypersensitivity (As classified by Gillam et al. 2000)

history and a thorough clinical and radiographic examination of the tooth in question, as well as, all adjacent teeth.

4.6 Induction of Pain of Dentin Hypersensitivity

Various methods and devices (Fig. 4.2) have been used to stimulate dentin hypersensitivity in the screening and assessment of severity in sufferers, but a suggestion has been made that at least two different stimuli should be used (Gernhardt 2013).

4.6.1 Tactile Method/Mechanical Stimulation

1. The simplest tactile method used to test for hypersensitivity is to lightly pass a sharp dental explorer over the sensitive area of a tooth and to grade the response of the patient on a severity scale, generally 0 to 3: 0, no pain felt; 1, slight pain or discomfort; 2, severe pain; and 3, severe pain that lasts.
2. *Mechanical Pressure Stimulators*. For example, the Smith and Ash (1964) scratch device is a device with a 15-mm (0.26-guage) stainless steel wire with a tip ground to a fine point and moveable across the highest arc of curvature of the facial surface of the sensitive tooth under test. The scratching force could be increased with a small screw that moves the tip closer to or away from the tooth surface.
3. Yeaple probe (1980). An electronic pressure-sensitive probe presented by Polson et al. (1980). The instrument consisted of a pen-like handpiece with a probe tip and an electronic control unit that allowed the probing force to be set at any level from 0.05 to 1 N. The allowable probing force was determined by an electromagnetic force that held an air gap shut until the preset probing force was reached, at which point the gap opened and a sound was produced. A variety of probing tips could be attached to the handpiece. Polson and his group used a 0.35-mm-diameter Hu-Friedy #26GL probe tip and set the probing force at 0.25 N (2.60 N/mm^2). Today, the probe is better known as the

"Yeaple probe" and is frequently used in studies of dentinal hypersensitivity (Kleinberg et al. 1990, 1994).

4. *Scratchometer*. It is a handheld scratch device (devised by Dr. Israel Kleinberg, University of Stony Brook, New York) and consists of a tension gauge and a sharp explorer-like probe that can be passed easily across a sensitive tooth. It has an indicator that is displaced by the arm of the explorer tine that records the force of displacement in centi-Newtons. The scratch process was reported with successively greater force in increments of 5 centi-Newtons (cN) until pain was felt. That force was considered the pain threshold for the teeth under test and was noted in centi-Newton.

4.6.2 Chemical (Osmotic) Stimuli (Gillam and Newman 1993)

This is the use of hypertonic solutions of glucose and sucrose, among others. The solution is applied with a cotton stick for 10 s, or until the subject reports discomfort. These solutions exert their effect through osmotic pressures that induce intratubular fluid movement. The use of this stimulus for the induction of dentin hypersensitivity is not advised due to the difficulty of controlling the patient's responses.

4.6.3 Electric Stimulation (Gillam and Newman 1993)

This is the gradual application of electric current to the dentinal surface. The risk posed by this method is the possibility of extending the stimulus to neighboring zones, due to current loss through the periodontium and subsequent stimulation of the periodontal nerves – thereby generating false-positive results.

1. *Pulp testers*: Pulp testers were used to quantify pain; however these were not useful for quantifying dentinal hypersensitivity because the increase in one unit on the pulp tester did not produce a linear increase in voltage.
2. *Dental pulp stethoscope*: A dental stethoscope composed of a measurement channel oscillator and a reference channel oscillator provided in combination. A measurement probe and a mouth mucosa lead element are respectively connected to the measurement channel oscillator, while at least one of equivalent circuits each consisting of an equivalent capacitor and an equivalent resistor connected in parallel to each other is selectively connected to the reference channel oscillator. The outputs of the measurement channel oscillator and reference channel oscillator are connected to the respective channels of a stereo headphone.

4.6.4 Dehydrating (Evaporative) Stimuli

1. *Cold air blast from a dental air syringe*: A simple thermal method for inducing tooth sensitivity is directing a burst of air at room temperature from a dental syringe onto the test tooth. Room air is cooler than the teeth, and cooling by this means can be easily detected as pain if the teeth are sensitive.
2. Also an air current from the dental chair can be applied for one second at a pressure of 45 psi and at an environmental temperature of 19–24 °C. The air current is applied at a distance of 1 cm and perpendicular to the surface of the tooth (Gillam et al. 2004; Addy et al. 2007). Application of the air current for more than one second leads to temperature variations. Due to the difficulty of localizing the sensitive dentin with the air current technique, the procedure is generally used to screen patients for dentin hypersensitivity.
3. *Yeh air thermal system*: An air thermal device devised by Dr. K.C. Yeh used a temperature-controlled stream of air as the stimulus. Air was heated to 100 F close to the temperature of the mouth. Its temp was then reduced until the subject felt pain or discomfort.
4. *Temptronic device (microprocessor temperature-controlled air delivery system)*: It is a device for determining the thermal sensitivity of teeth and other nerve-sensitive

tissue. The device comprises a portable probe for emitting a stream of pressurized fluid and a temperature controller for controlling the temperature of the emitted fluid.

4.6.5 Thermal Stimulation

1. *Cold water testing*: Another method of stimulation is the application of water at a temperature of 7 °C (Gillam and Newman 1993). A battery of syringes containing water at different temperatures (between 0 and 20 °C) – beginning with the warmest water and gradually to lower temperatures – may be employed. Application to the tooth should not exceed 3 s, and if no response is obtained, 3 min should be allowed to elapse before continuing with the next test at a lower temperature. The temperature of the water is lowered in steps of 5 °C, and testing is stopped when a painful response is recorded or when 0 °C is reached (nonsensitive tooth).
2. Heat testing can be undertaken using a stick of heated gutta-percha or hot water. A gutta-percha stick, preferably base-plate gutta-percha, is heated with a naked flame or an electric heater until it becomes soft and glistens. It is then applied to the Vaseline-coated surface of the test tooth. This test may be difficult to use on the posterior teeth because of limited access and vision. Conversely, insufficient heating of the gutta-percha stick could result in the stimulus being too weak to elicit a response. Hot water can also be administered through an irrigating syringe; this must be performed under rubber dam isolation.
3. *Electronic threshold measurement device*: The apparatus consisted of a miniature thermistor connected to a medical multichannel recorder with a handheld event recorder. The thermistor was placed adjacent to the hypersensitive area for an accurate temperature measure of the point at which the subject first reported pain (Thrash et al. 1983).
4. *Thermoelectric device*: The device includes a handle having a thermally and electrically conductive probe tip, a heat sink within the handle, and a thermoelectric element having a first junction thermally coupled to the probe tip and a second junction thermally coupled to the heat sink. Heating or cooling of the probe tip is accomplished by passage of electric current through the thermoelectric element. A temperature-sensing device such as a thermistor is thermally coupled to the probe tip, and temperature regulation circuitry responsive to the state of the temperature-sensing element regulates the current to the thermoelectric element to maintain the temperature of the probe tip constant at a predetermined desired value.
5. *Ethyl chloride*: This can be sprayed onto a cotton pledget and placed against the suspected sensitive surface.
6. *Ice stick*: A simple means of applying a cold stimulus to a tooth is to wrap a sliver of ice in wet gauze and place it against the suspected sensitive surface.

4.6.6 Are There Radiographic Changes Associating with Hypersensitive Teeth?

Generally with dentin hypersensitivity, radiographic changes do not appear in the bone. A shallow carious lesion may be visible but there will not be any widening of the periodontal ligament space or thickening of the bone around the apex. If these types of changes are present, then the hypersensitivity has probably progressed into irreversible pulpitis, a situation that may need other treatment approaches. In severe cases of cervical erosion or abrasion, it is possible to see loss of tooth density in the cervical zone.

Conclusion

Correct diagnosis is extremely important since the history may be clinically confounded with other clinical conditions. It requires adequate knowledge of the underlying etiology and a correct differential diagnosis with respect to other dental processes that can be accompanied by brief and acute pain. As limited equipment can be employed in the diagnosis of dentin hypersensitivity, clinicians must be familiar with several of the factors discussed in this chapter, i.e., characteristics of the pain, age of occurrence, tooth predilection, side and site predilection, and history of interaction with predisposing factors. Taking these factors into consideration, it is necessary to exclude other forms of pain or dental sensitivity.

References

Addy M, West NX, Barlow A et al (2007) Dentin hypersensitivity: is there both stimulus and placebo responses in clinical trials. Int J Dent Hyg 5(1):53–59

Anderson DJ, Matthews B, Shelton LE (1967) Variations in the sensitivity to osmotic stimulation of human dentin. Arch Oral Biol 12(1):43–47

Andrej MK (2002) Dentin hypersensitivity: simple steps for everyday diagnosis and management. Int Dent J 52:394–396

Andrew D, Matthews B (2000) Displacement of the contents of dentinal tubules and sensory transduction in intradental nerves of the cat. J Physiol 529 (Pt 3):791–802

Bamise CT, Olusile AO, Oginni AO et al (2007) Prevalence of dentin hypersensitivity among adult patients attending a Nigerian teaching hospital. Oral Health Prev Dent 5(1):49–53

Bender IB (2000) Pulpal pain diagnosis—a review. J Endod 26(3):175–179

Braennstroem M, Astroem A (1964) A study on the mechanism of pain elicited from the dentin. J Dent Res 43:619–625

Brannstrom M, Astrom A (1972) The hydrodynamics of the dentin; its possible relationship to dental pain. Int Dent J 22:219–227

Canadian Advisory Board on Dentin Hypersensitivity (2003) Consensus-based recommendations for the diagnosis and management of dentin hypersensitivity. J Can Dent Assoc 69:221–226

Curro FA (1990) Tooth hypersensitivity in the spectrum of pain. Dent Clin North Am 34:429–437

Dababneh RH, Khouri AT, Addy M (1999) Dentin hypersensitivity an enigma? A review of terminology, epidemiology, mechanisms, aetiology and management. Br Dent J 187:606–611

Drisko CH (2002) Dentin hypersensitivity – dental hygiene and periodontal considerations. Int Dent J 52:385–393

Gernhardt CR (2013) How valid and applicable are current diagnostic criteria and assessment methods for dentin hypersensitivity? An overview. Clin Oral Investig 17(Suppl 1):31–40

Gillam DG, Newman HN (1993) Assessment of pain in cervical dentinal sensitivity studies. A review. J Clin Periodontol 20(6):383–394

Gillam DG, Orchardson R, Närhi MVO, Kontturi-Närhi V (2000) Present and future methods for the evaluation of pain associated with dentin hypersensitivity. In: Addy M, Embery G, Edgar WM, Orchardson R (eds) Tooth wear and sensitivity. Martin Dunitz, London, pp 283–297

Gillam DG, Newman HN, Davies EH et al (2004) Clinical evaluation of ferric oxalate in relieving dentin hypersensitivity. J Oral Rehabil 31(3):245–250

Gunji T (1982) Morphological research on the sensitivity of dentin. Arch Histol Jpn 45:45–67

Holland GR (1981) The incidence of dentinal tubules containing more than one process in the cuspal dentin of cat canine teeth. Anat Rec 200:437–442

Holland GR, Narhi MN, Addy M et al (1997) Guidelines for the design and conduct of clinical trials on dentin hypersensitivity. J Clin Periodontol 24(11):808–813

Irwin CR, McCusker P (1997) Prevalence of dentin hypersensitivity in general dental population. J Ir Dent Assoc 43:7–9

Kleinberg I, Kaufman HW, Confessore F (1990) Methods of measuring tooth hypersensitivity. Dent Clin North Am 34:515–529

Kleinberg I, Kaufman HW, Wolff M (1994) Measurement of tooth hypersensitivity and oral factors involved in its development. Arch Oral Biol 39:63S–71S

Lilja J (1980) Sensory differences between crown and root dentin in human teeth. Acta Odontol Scand 38:285–291

Matthews B, Vongsavan N (1994) Interactions between neural and hydrodynamic mechanisms in dentin and pulp. Arch Oral Biol 39(Suppl):87S–95S

Narhi MV (1985) Dentin sensitivity: a review. J Biol Buccale 13(2):75–96

Narhi MV, Hirvonen T (1987) The response of dog intradental nerves to hypertonic solutions of CaCl2 and NaCl, and other stimuli, applied to exposed dentin. Arch Oral Biol 32(11):781–786

Narhi MV, Hirvonen TJ, Hakumäki MOK (1982a) Responses of intradental nerve fibres to stimulation of dentin and pulp. Acta Physiol Scand 115(2): 173–178

Narhi M, Jyvasjarvi E, Hirvonen T et al (1982b) Activation of heat-sensitive nerve fibres in the dental pulp of the cat. Pain 14(4):317–326

Narhi M, Jyvasjarvi E, Virtanen A et al (1992a) Role of intradental A- and C-type nerve fibres in dental pain mechanisms. Proc Finn Dent Soc 88(Suppl 1):507–516

Narhi M, Kontturi-Narhi V, Hirvonen T et al (1992b) Neurophysiological mechanisms of dentin hypersensitivity. Proc Finn Dent Soc 88(Suppl 1):15–22

Olgart L, Kerezoudis NP (1994) Nerve pulp interactions. Archs Oral Biol 39:47s–54s

Orchardson R, Collins WJ (1987a) Thresholds of hypersensitive teeth to 2 forms of controlled stimulation. J Clin Periodontol 14(2):68–73

Orchardson R, Collins WJN (1987b) Clinical features of hypersensitive teeth. Br Dent J 162:253–256

Pashley DH (1986) Sensitivity of dentin to chemical stimuli. Endod Dent Traumatol 2(4):130–137

Pashley DH (1990) Mechanisms of dentin sensitivity. Dent Clin North Am 34(3):449–473
Polson AM, Caton IB, Yeaple RN et al (1980) Histological determination of probe tip penetration into gingival sulcus of humans using an electronic pressure sensitive probe. J Clin Periodontol 7(6):479–488
Rees JS (2000) The prevalence of dentin hypersensitivity in general dental practice in the UK. J Clin Periodontol 27(11):860–865
Schuurs AHB, Wesselink PR, Eijkman MAJ et al (1995) Dentist's views on cervical hypersensitivity and their knowledge of its treatment. Endod Dent Traumatol 1:240–244
Smith BA, Ash MM Jr (1964) Evaluation of a desensitizing dentifrice and cervical hypersensitivity. J Am Dent Assoc 68:639–647
Taani SD, Awartani F (2002) Clinical evaluation of cervical dentin hypersensitivity (CDS) in patients attending general dental clinics (PDC) and periodontal specialty clinics (PSC). J Clin Periodontol 29:118–122
Ten Cate AR (1994) Oral histology, development structure and function. CV Mosby Year book, St Louis
Thrash WJ, Dorman HL, Smith FD (1983) A method to measure pain associated with hypersensitive dentin. J Periodontol 54(3):160–162
Trowbridge HO (1985) Intradental sensory units: physiological and clinical aspects. J Endod 11(11):489–498
Trowbridge HO (2003) Pulp biology: progress during the past 25 years. Aust Endod J 29(1):5–12
Trowbridge HO, Franks M, Korostoff E et al (1980) Sensory response to thermal stimulation in human teeth. J Endod 6(1):405–412
Vongsavan N, Matthews B (2007) The relationship between the discharge of interdental nerves and the rate of fluid flow through dentin in the cat. Arch Oral Biol 52(7):640–647, Epub 2007 Feb 15

Treatment Approaches for Dentin Hypersensitivity

5

David G. Gillam

Abstract

The aim of this chapter is to review the various treatment approaches used by clinicians to treat dentin hypersensitivity and evaluate their efficacy in reducing dentin hypersensitivity. Evidence from both in vitro and in vivo studies will be assessed to determine whether there is any support for these treatment products and procedures based on their proposed underlying mechanism of action.

5.1 Introduction

The hydrodynamic theory promotes two basic approaches based on in vitro, in situ, animal and human studies for treating dentin hypersensitivity (DH) (Ling and Gillam 1996; Orchardson and Gillam 2006) (Fig. 5.1):

1. Dentin blocking agents that occlude patent (open) tubules (fluoride, strontium salts, oxalate, calcium phosphate, restorative materials, etc.) and as a consequence reduce any stimulus-evoked fluid movements within the dentin tubule
2. Nerve desensitisation agents that reduce intradental nerve excitability (e.g. potassium ions, guanethidine) in order to prevent a response from intradental nerves to the stimulus-evoked fluid movements within the dentin tubules

It should be acknowledged that in vitro results demonstrating superiority of the various products under examination should not be extrapolated into making claims on the efficacy of these products without first undergoing extensive clinical evaluation. There are however a vast array of products currently out on the commercial market with various claims of clinical efficacy in reducing DH, although currently there does not appear to be a gold standard product or therapy universally accepted by clinicians to treat the condition (see Chap. 6).

Application of these successfully tested products may either involve 'in-office' procedures by a clinician using a restorative approach (for example, restorative materials in the form of dentin bonding agents, glass ionomer cements (GIC), and periodontal surgical techniques) or by a clinician recommending an over-the-counter (OTC) approach (involving toothpastes, gels, mouthwashes).

5.2 Dentin Blocking Agents

Currently the hydrodynamic theory (Brännström 1963) is generally considered to be the mechanism of choice although other alternative mechanisms of stimulus transmission cannot be ruled

D.G. Gillam
Centre for Adult Oral Health, Institute of Dentistry, Barts and the London School of Medicine and Dentistry QMUL, Turner Street, London E1 2AD, UK
e-mail: d.g.gillam@qmul.ac.uk

S. Taha, B.H. Clarkson (eds.), *Clinician's Guide to the Diagnosis and Management of Tooth Sensitivity*,
DOI 10.1007/978-3-642-45164-5_5, © Springer-Verlag Berlin Heidelberg 2014

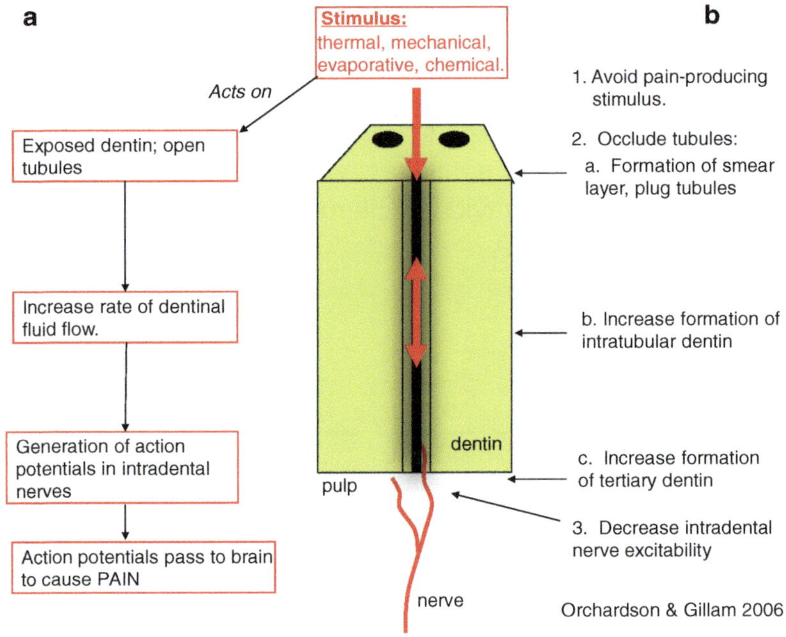

Fig. 5.1 Outline of the hydrodynamic mechanism by which (**a**) stimuli activate intradental nerves to cause pain and (**b**) subsequent resolution following natural desensitisation and treatment (Acknowledgement Orchardson and Gillam 2006)

out, since some clinical phenomena cannot be explained solely by this theory (Gillam 1992; Orchardson and Gillam 2006) (Fig. 5.1).

There are a number of products commercially available for the treatment of DH these include both in-office applied and over-the-counter products. The proposed mode of action for most of these products has been established using in vitro, animal, in situ and in vivo studies (Orchardson and Gillam 2006 Tables 5.1a and 5.1b).

5.2.1 Strontium-Containing Toothpastes

Strontium chloride has been claimed to act as both a protein precipitant and a tubule-occluding agent (Cohen 1961; Skurnik 1963; Blitzer 1967; Gedalia et al. 1978; Uchida et al. 1980). Gutentag (1965) however also demonstrated that strontium may stabilise excitable neural membranes by modifying their permeability to sodium and potassium. Several investigators have shown that strontium ions may be deposited as an insoluble barrier, possibly a calcium strontium–hydroxyapatite complex, at the dentin tubule openings (Pawlowska 1956; Ross 1961; Blitzer 1967; Gedalia et al. 1978). Kun (1976) however demonstrated in vitro that a topical application of concentrated strontium chloride solution produced a continuous deposit on the dentin surface as well as a degree of penetration into the dentin tubules. Furthermore he proposed as a result of evidence from the electron probe microanalysis and X-ray diffraction studies that the fundamental mechanism of the formation of strontium deposits was an exchange with the calcium of the dentin, resulting in recrystallisation in the form of strontium apatite. Evidence from other in vitro studies (Greenhill and Pashley 1981; Mostafa et al. 1983; Pashley et al. 1984; Addy et al. 1991), however, would appear to suggest that these results were attributable not to active ingredient per se but to the abrasive component(s) of a toothpaste which may contribute to the formation of a smear layer and to some degree occlude or block the exposed dentin tubule opening (Mordan et al. 2002) (Fig. 5.2a, b).

5.2.2 Selected Calcium Compounds

5.2.2.1 Casein Phosphopeptide–Amorphous Calcium Phosphate (CPP–ACP)

Toothpastes containing Casein Phosphopeptide–Amorphous Calcium Phosphate (CPP–ACP) were primarily developed for anticaries and

Table 5.1a Characteristics of selected occluding toothpastes

Product	Composition	Proposed mode of action
SensiStat®	Contains arginine in combination with calcium and bicarbonate/ carbonate	The arginine complex binds to the tooth surface and allows the calcium carbonate to slowly dissolve and release calcium. Limited in vitro and in vivo studies have been published in support of both laboratory and clinical claims for the product. Tubular occlusion
Colgate Pro-Argin™	Hydroxyapatite, sodium monofluorophosphate (MFP)	Recent in vitro and in vivo studies have been published in support of both laboratory and clinical claims for the product. Tubule occlusion
SensiShield® (NovaMin®)	Composed of calcium phosphorus, sodium and silica (calcium sodium phosphosilicate)	NovaMin® in contact with saliva and water reacts and releases Ca and PO4 ions. Sodium ions in the NovaMin particles exchange with hydrogen cations which in turn allows the calcium and phosphate ions to be released. A calcium phosphate layer is formed and subsequently crystallises into hydroxycarbonate apatite. The exposed dentin surface appears to act as a nucleation site for these ions to form hydroxycarbonate apatite and bypasses the intermediate phase of ACP formation. Mainly in vitro support for occlusion of dentine tubules, limited published clinical data supporting clinical efficacy of the product. Tubular occlusion
Amorphous calcium phosphate (ACP)	ACP is inorganic in nature and is made by combining soluble salts of calcium and phosphate through a two-phase system containing Ca in one part and PO4 in another. When mixed together they react to form an amorphous phosphate material that precipitates on to the tooth surface	ACP is highly soluble and susceptible to acid attack, and as such the ACP is not protected and as it has no delivery system, it has lower substantivity. It has lower substantivity. ACP is not bioavailable after the product is rinsed away. Previously incorporated in Enamelon toothpaste (no longer available) which relied on a dual-chamber system in the toothpaste tube. The product is now available in Enamel Care toothpaste (Church and Dwight). Limited and equivocal published data for effectiveness of ACP in the treatment of dentin hypersensitivity
Recaldent (CPP–ACP)	Casein phosphates (CPP) are peptides derived from milk protein casein that are complexed with calcium (Ca) and phosphate (PO4). In this complex the CPP maintains the Ca and PO4 ions in an amorphous form (ACP). The milk-derived peptide containing amorphous Ca and PO4 is the driving mechanism that binds to plaque, bacteria and the tooth surface	CPP–ACP uses peptides derived from the milk protein casein to maintain Ca and PO_4 in an amorphous calcium phosphate. The CPP binds to surfaces such as plaque, bacteria and soft tissue providing a bioavailable Ca and PO_4 at the surface of the tooth without precipitation. The ACP is released during acidic challenges. Stabilisation of ACP by the CPP ensures the delivery of Ca and PO_4 ions into the tooth structure before the ions crystallise. Most in vitro and in vivo studies support the product's anticaries benefit, however there does not appear to be any published clinical support on its effect in reducing dentin hypersensitivity
Nanit®active (Henkel)	Hydroxyapatite, sodium monofluorophosphate (MFP)	According to Henkel's product literature Nanit®active induces a process referred to as neomineralisation. The Nanit®active nanoparticles react with the calcium and phosphate ions in saliva, and a new protective layer is formed on the tooth surface (1–2 μm). Limited data available at present. Tubular occlusion

Acknowledgement from Mason et al. (2010) modified

remineralisation strategies rather than for the treatment of DH per se. According to Reynolds (1998), the CPP component binds to surfaces in the oral environment such as plaque, bacteria and soft tissue providing a bioavailable Ca and PO_4 at the surface of the tooth (e.g. enamel) without any precipitation. The ACP is subsequently released from the dental plaque during acidic challenges. The stabilisation of ACP component by the CPP ensures the delivery of both Ca and PO_4 ions onto the enamel surface for remineralisation. Both in vitro and in vivo studies have demonstrated that

Table 5.1b Characteristics of selected dentin blocking toothpastes

Product	Composition	Proposed mode of action
Blanx® Biorepair®	Hydroxyapatite, sodium monofluorophosphate (MFP)	Limited published data available at present. Tubular occlusion
Strontium salts (Sensodyne)	Strontium chloride (original), no fluoride	Hydrated technology. Published in vitro and in vivo studies supporting both the proposed mode of action and clinical effectiveness of both the acetate and chloride variants of the product. Tubular occlusion
	Strontium actate, sodium monofluorophosphate (MFP)	
Stannous fluoride	Stannous fluoride	Anhydrous technology. Uses hexametaphosphate to limit stains associated with the use of stannous ions. Two clinical studies in support of claims. Tubular occlusion
Crest® ProHealth™		
Colgate SnF_2	Stannous fluoride, potassium nitrate (5 %)	Dual-chamber delivery system. Published in vitro and in vivo studies supporting both the proposed mode of action and clinical effectiveness of the product. Presence of potassium would indicate its use as a nerve desensitiser; however in vitro studies tubule occlusion is in evidence. According to Mason et al. (2010) this product is no longer commercially available
Amine fluoride (elmex SENSITIVE)	Amine fluoride (olaflur)	Amine fluoride leads to the formation of a protective layer on the dentin containing calcium fluoride, which helps promote remineralisation and tubular occlusion. Limited published data available. Tubular occlusion

Acknowledgement from Mason et al. (2010) modified

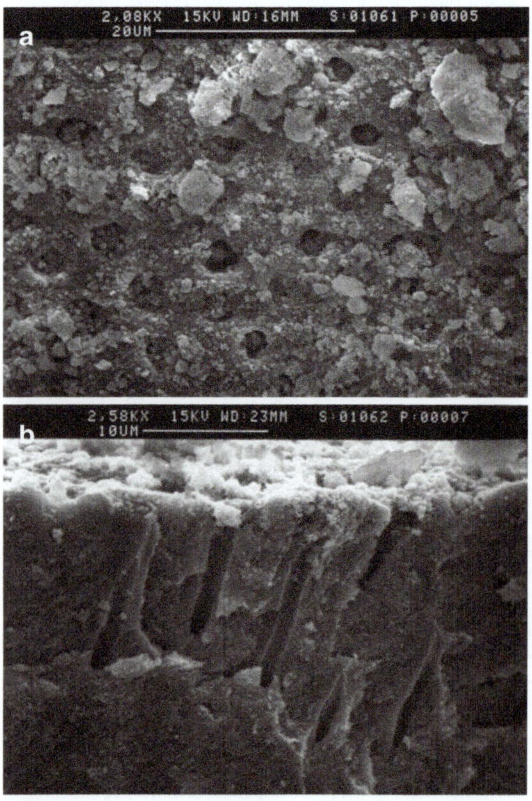

Fig. 5.2 (**a**) Coverage of the exposed dentin following a 2 min application of a fluoride toothpaste (Mordan et al. 2002). (**b**) Evidence of tubular occlusion of dentin tubules by toothpaste ingredients (e.g., silica) following a 2 min application of a fluoride toothpaste (Mordan et al. 2002)

calcium phosphate preparations deposit a mineral precipitate on to the dentin surface, block dentin tubules and reduce dentin permeability in the dentin disc model and DH in patients (Ebisu 2002; Suge et al. 2002; Cherng et al. 2004; Geiger et al. 2003; Azarpazhooh and Limeback 2008; Charig et al. 2009; Gandolfi et al. 2010; Walsh 2010) (Table 5.1a).

5.2.2.2 Calcium Carbonate and Arginine (Colgate Pro-Argin™)

Kleinberg (2002) suggested at physiological pH the positively charged arginine in the arginine/insoluble calcium carbonate compound combination binds to the negatively charged dentin surface enabling a calcium-rich mineral layer into the open (exposed) dentin tubule to act as an effective plug or tubular occludent. Initial laboratory (in vitro) evidence appears to support this in that the product does occlude the dentin tubules and effectively block fluid flow and is resistant to an acid challenge (Petrou et al. 2009), and subsequent clinical studies evidence appears to support its efficacy as a desensitiser (Ayad et al. 2009; Docimo et al. 2009; Hamlin et al. 2009; Nathoo et al. 2009; Schiff et al. 2009a, b, 2011; Que et al. 2010; Cummins 2011) (Table 5.1a). Recent systematic reviews by Sharif et al. (2013) and Yan et al. (2013) have also indicated that there are clinical benefits for using Pro-Argin™ toothpastes in reducing DH; however both these investigators raised concerns regarding the quality of the conducted studies and recommended that further well-designed studies should be conducted to determine the efficacy of the product in reducing DH.

5.2.2.3 Bioactive Glasses

Bioactive glasses (calcium sodium phosphosilicate), for example, NovaMin® (developed by NovaMin Technology Inc., Alachua, FL, USA) based on the original 45S5 Bioglass® formulation by Larry Hench (US Biomaterials Corp., Jacksonville, FL, USA, now GSK) (Hench 2006), have been incorporated into toothpastes for the treatment of DH. The proposed mode of action is by the precipitating of hydroxycarbonate apatite (HCA) onto the dentin surface and subsequently occluding the dentin tubules (Litkowski et al. 1998; Gillam et al. 2002; Tai et al. 2006; Vollenweider et al. 2007; Burwell 2006; Burwell et al. 2009; Wang et al. 2010; Pradeep and Sharma 2010; Mneimne et al. 2011) (Table 5.1a).

One advantage of the precipitated HCA layer is that it is chemically and structurally similar to natural enamel and dentin (Burwell 2006). A recent randomised double-blind controlled trial, by Orsini et al. (2010), compared the clinical efficacy of a new toothpaste containing (HCA) nanocrystals and a sodium fluoride/potassium nitrate toothpaste and concluded that a new novel toothpaste formulation containing zinc-HCA nanocrystals significantly reduced DH after 4 and 8 weeks. There have however been concerns over the long-term durability of HCA in the oral environment, and it has been postulated that the formation of fluorapatite (FAp) rather than HCA is preferable, since this layer may be more resistant to acid attack and would therefore dissolve less readily when teeth are exposed to acidic conditions (e.g. during consumption of fruit juice and carbonated beverages). It has been recently demonstrated that fluoride-containing bioactive glasses form FAp rather than HCA in physiological solutions (Brauer et al. 2010).

5.2.2.4 Hydroxyapatite-Based Toothpastes

According to Hill et al. (2012), hydroxyapatite-based toothpastes have been widely used in China and the Far East (Park et al. 2005; Kang et al. 2009; Kim et al. 2009; Yuan et al. 2012). The published literature on hydroxyapatite toothpastes however is mainly in non-English journals and may, therefore, not be readily available in an English translation format (Park et al. 2005; Kang et al. 2009; Kim et al. 2009; Yuan et al. 2012). More recently, the commercial emphasis has focused on the use of nanocrystalline hydroxyapatite in toothpastes for desensitising and remineralising strategies (Rimondini et al. 2007; Orsini et al. 2010; Tschoppe et al. 2011). The proposed mechanism of action for hydroxyapatite-containing toothpastes is blocking the dentin tubules (Rimondini et al. 2007; Hill et al. 2012; Yuan et al. 2012) (Table 5.1a).

5.2.3 Selected Fluoride Formulations

Fluoride was first proposed as a desensitising agent in 1941 by Lukomsky (1941) and has subsequently used in toothpastes, gels, mouth rinses and varnishes (Orchardson and Gillam 2006). Sodium fluoride and stannous fluoride have been shown to reduce DH (Morris et al. 1999), and amine fluoride has also been incorporated into dentifrices although there is currently limited published data to support its use. Stannous fluoride (SnF_2) in a 0.4 % glycerin gel has also been reported to be effective in reducing DH (Miller et al. 1969) although this formulation and the use of SnF_2 may be problematic for a number of reasons, for example, (1) when placed in an aqueous environment, it appears to undergo hydrolysis and precipitates out of solution (Miller et al. 1969) hence the incorporation into a gel and (2) poor taste and staining characteristics. More recently investigators have demonstrated that a reformulated toothpaste containing stannous fluoride with a novel 0.454 % stabilised stannous fluoride formulation containing sodium hexametaphosphate (SHMP) was effective in reducing DH during an 8-week treatment compared to a sodium fluoride toothpaste as a control (Schiff et al. 2005, 2006; Day et al. 2010; Einwag et al. 2010; cited by Ni et al. 2010). According to Greenhill and Pashley (1981), fluorides decrease the permeability of dentine in vitro possibly by the precipitation of insoluble calcium fluoride within the tubules. However the exact mechanism whereby fluoride reduces DH is unknown. Fluoride incorporation increases the resistance of dentin to decalcification (Furseth 1970) and reduces its solubility (Sandoval and Shannon 1969) as fluorapatite is more resistant to acid attack(s) than hydroxyapatite. Sodium monofluorophosphate has also been previously investigated as a toothpaste ingredient with desensitising effects by Hazen et al. (1968) and by Addy et al. (1987) who reported on its clinical effectiveness in combination with strontium acetate. Recently several investigators have reported on the clinical efficacy of a combined sodium monofluorophosphate/strontium acetate formulation for the treatment of DH (Mason et al. 2010; Hughes et al. 2010) (Table 5.1b). Higher fluoride concentration toothpastes containing 2,800/5,000 ppm sodium fluoride (Colgate Duraphat) have also been advocated for prevention of dental caries and as such may be of potential benefit in the treatment of root caries and DH.

One however should not ignore that natural desensitisation of dentin (both internally and externally) may occur irrespective of whatever treatment is provided by the clinician to the patient. For example, Orchardson and Gillam (2006) have suggested that there may be natural desensitising of dentin through precipitation of salivary proteins, toothpaste ingredients, etc., forming a smear layer which may occlude the dentin tubules or remineralisation (Pashley 1992a; Kawasaki et al. 2001) as well as the formation of both intra-tubular dentin and secondary/tertiary dentin over time (Addy and Dowell 1983) (Fig. 5.1).

5.3 Nerve Desensitisation and Noci0ception

As indicated earlier, the hydrodynamic theory (Brännström 1963) is generally considered to be the mechanism of choice, and as with dentin blocking agents, this theory appears to explain how nerve desensitisation may occur following the application of potassium-containing products (e.g. toothpastes gels, mouth rinses).

Several investigators (Greenhill and Pashley 1981; Pashley et al. 1984) however failed to observe any effect of potassium nitrate (either as a 30 % solution or 5 % toothpaste) in terms of a reduction in dentin fluid flow (dentin permeability) in the in vitro dentin disc model. In other words, these investigators were unable to demonstrate whether potassium nitrate reduced DH by blocking the dentin tubules and were therefore unable to determine the exact mechanism of action of potassium-containing toothpastes which were reported to be clinically effective when treating DH. These investigators however did not rule out the possibility that these agents may desensitise dentin via neural effects unrelated to hydrodynamic mechanisms.

In order to ascertain the precise mechanism for action for potassium, several investigators utilised a neurophysiological animal (cat) model which involved deep-cut cavity preparations with a very thin slice of dentin between the exposed dentin surface and the pulp (Kim 1986; Markowitz and Kim 1985, 1990; Markowitz et al. 1991). These investigators subsequently demonstrated that when using large molar concentrations of various divalent cation solutions (including potassium) applied to the dentin surface, both intradental nerve activity and sensory nerve activity were reduced. It was also evident from these studies that the important chemical moiety of potassium nitrate was the potassium salt and not the nitrate anion as previously believed. Furthermore potassium appeared to be the more effective desensitising agent compared to the other solutions tested irrespective of which combination of anion was used. On the basis of these observations, these investigators proposed that the mode of potassium desensitisation was through raising the intra-tubular potassium (K^+)

Table 5.2 Characteristics of selected nerve depolarising toothpastes

Product	Composition	Proposed mode of action
Sensodyne	Potassium nitrate, sodium fluoride (NaF)	Hydrated toothpaste technology. Evidence of a desensitising action based on historical animal studies. No evidence of tubular occlusion when potassium ions were tested in vitro. Evidence from the published literature suggests that potassium-containing toothpastes are effective in reducing dentin hypersensitivity although there is no evidence to suggest that it is by nerve depolarisation. Recent clinical study has reported that there is a transient depolarising effect when potassium ions are applied on exposed dentin
Colgate	Potassium nitrate, sodium monofluorophosphate (MFP)	
Crest	Potassium sodium fluoride (NaF)	
Sensodyne	Potassium chloride sodium fluoride (NaF)	
Colgate	Potassium citrate sodium monofluorophosphate (MFP)	

Acknowledgement from Mason et al. (2010)

concentration which would render the intradental nerves less excitable to any further stimulation by depolarisation of the nerve fibre membrane. Initially this increase in the potassium ion content elicits an increased number of action potentials, after the initial depolarisation; however the nerve fibre(s) cannot depolarise due to the maintained high levels of extracellular potassium ion content and as a consequence a sustained depolarised state occurs (axonal accommodation).

The interpretation based on the investigation by Kim and co-workers (1985, 1986, 1990, 1991 see above) has however been criticised by Sena (1990) who suggested that as a result of the deep-cut cavity preparations in the cat, the applied potassium ion only had a short distance to traverse the length of the dentin tubule to exert its effect to desensitise the nerve. In the normal clinical situation (in intact human teeth), however, the incoming potassium ion (e.g. if applied in a toothpaste product on the exposed cervical dentin) would have to overcome the opposing pulpal pressure that produces an outward flow of dentin fluid. Such an outward flow may therefore prevent the inward diffusion of substances from the oral cavity. Currently it is important to note that this proposed mechanism was based on animals and has not been confirmed for human dentin (Orchardson and Gillam 2000) (Table 5.2). For example if the desensitising effects of potassium are due to action potential inactivation, one might expect as Orchardson and Gillam (2000) suggested that the patient would experience a transient pain when a potassium-containing toothpaste is applied to the exposed dentin surface. This phenomenon has not been reported for toothpastes in humans. It may also be of note in this context, however, to reconsider the work by Anderson and co-workers (1958, 1962a, b) who postulated that if dentin was directly innervated, then chemical stimuli to the exposed dentin surface should cause a patient discomfort. Application of algogenic (pain-inducing) substances such as potassium chloride, acetylcholine and histamine, however, failed to elicit a response. By way of contrast when these substances were applied directly to exposed pulpal tissue, an immediate response was elicited (Anderson and Naylor 1962; Anderson 1968, 1972). This observation may therefore be of interest when ascertaining the precise mode of action of potassium-containing preparations.

Several investigators have however attempted to explain the role of potassium diffusion across dentin (Stead et al. 1996; McCormack and Davies 1996).

(a) *Mathematical Model of Potassium Ion Diffusion*

In order to ascertain whether the potassium ion could diffuse down the dentin tubule, Stead et al. (1996) proposed a mathematical model of potassium ion diffusion which incorporated a number of variables, for example, dentin thickness, tubule diameter, time, diffusion gradient, outward fluid flow, the constituents of dentin fluid (molecule size), permeability of the odontoblast layer and the concentration of potassium (based on 5 % potassium in toothpastes).

According to these investigators, the application of potassium-containing preparations to the exposed dentin may increase potassium ions at the inner ends of the dentinal tubules to levels sufficient to inactivate intradental nerves; however, the localised increase in potassium ions may only be transient, and the concentration change will also be reduced by conditions that increase the tubular fluid flow velocity or the permeability of the barrier between the tubule and the pulp. The prediction from this model regarding nature of the transient effect of the potassium ion on nerve inactivation may be of interest particularly in the light of the results from the clinical studies by Ajcharanukul et al. (2007, 2011, 2012). These investigators utilised a cut cavity preparation approach based on the animal model in human subjects and demonstrated that potassium salts had a transient desensitising effect as predicted by Stead et al. (1996). However one of the conclusions from these studies was that the hydrodynamic mechanism responsible for responses to stimulation of dentin in humans has different properties from those demonstrated in the cat and may not necessarily be mediated by a hydrodynamic mechanism.

(b) *The Role of Nitric Oxide as a Secondary Messenger*

One of the problems with the mathematical model of potassium diffusion as proposed by Stead et al. (1996) was the various constraints to the diffusion of the potassium ion along the entire length of the dentin tubule (Orchardson and Gillam 2000). An alternative mechanism for potassium ion-mediated desensitisation was proposed by McCormack and Davies (1996). These investigators suggested that the potassium ion could evoke a novel synthesis of a mobile secondary messenger (nitric oxide) within dentin and the dental pulp. The proposed hypothesis is that the potassium ion may act on the odontoblast process to release nitric oxide (in the dental pulp) which in turn produces an analgesic effect by modulating nociceptive input through downregulation of sensitised nociceptors. Although this hypothesis may provide a plausible explanation for the role of the potassium ion in the treatment of DH there does not appear to be any supporting evidence from the published literature (Orchardson and Gillam 2000; Jackson 2000).

According to Orchardson and Gillam (2000), there appears to be no convincing evidence that desensitising preparations based on potassium chloride, nitrate and citrate act in the manner proposed. It is possible that any desensitising effects may be due to constituents other than the potassium salts. Although there is some evidence that toothpastes containing potassium ions are more effective than minus-active preparations in reducing dentin hypersensitivity, the potassium-containing preparations are not always superior to controls such as sodium monofluorophosphate. Furthermore while a number of studies included in the Orchardson and Gillam (2000) review reported that potassium-containing salts were significantly better than the inactive (placebo) controls, a number of these studies did report an appreciable reduction in dentin hypersensitivity with the supposedly 'inactive' controls. One of the problems, in evaluating the various studies was the reported variation(s) in the extent of the 'control/placebo' response which may have accounted for most of the disparities between trial outcomes (Jackson 2000; Cummins 2009, 2010). A previous published systematic review by Poulsen et al. (2006) included six studies in the meta-analysis and concluded that there was no clear evidence available in the published literature for the support of potassium-containing toothpastes for the relief of DH. More recent reviews by Pol et al. (2010) and Karim and Gillam (2013) also highlighted the lack of data on the efficacy of potassium salts in reducing dentin hypersensitivity.

The use of topical guanethidine (1 % guanethidine solution (Ismelin, Ciba-Geigy, UK)) as a desensitiser has also been advocated although there are only two published studies by Hannington-Kiff and Dunne (1993) and Dunne and Hannington-Kiff (1993). These investigators proposed that topically applied guanethidine affects the anti-noradrenergic mechanisms in the teeth.

5.4 Placebo Effect

Both placebo and nocebo effects have been documented in the published literature and may impact on the results from studies evaluating the efficacy of a drug. The term 'nocebo' comes from the Latin 'noceo', to harm, and means 'I shall harm', whereas the term 'placebo' means 'I shall please' (Definition of placebo 2013: http://www.medterms.com). A negative placebo effect may occur during a clinical study where patients participating in the study experience adverse side effects unrelated to the specific pharmacological action of the drug that they are taking. The nocebo effect may be associated with a subject's prior expectations of adverse effects from treatment as well as with conditioning in which the subject learns from prior experiences to associate a medication with certain somatic symptoms (Definition of nocebo effect 2013: http://www.medterms.com). The placebo or placebo effect has been defined in the following manner:

(a) A substance containing no medication and prescribed or given to reinforce a patient's expectation to get well.
(b) An inactive substance or preparation used as a control in an experiment or test to determine the effectiveness of a medicinal drug.
(c) An active placebo – a placebo used in experimental tests of a drug that has noticeable side effects; 'an active placebo mimics the side effects of the experimental drug' (Definition of active placebo 2013: www.thefreedictionary.com).

According to Oken (2008), the interaction between the clinician and the subject during a clinical study may have an impact on outcomes independent of any specific treatment. For example, 'expectancy' may be affected by the personal history of subject–clinician interactions and shared experiences of the subject and clinician. Several investigators have also suggested that any placebo effects during a study may also be influenced by the number of subject–clinician interactions (Ilnyckyj et al. 1997; Paternak and Zimmerman 2007 cited by Oken 2008). There may also be other non-specific benefits from this interaction during a clinical study, for example, stress reduction, decreased anxiety or improvement of mood of the subject. According to Oken (2008), some clinicians are perceived to be better clinicians than others as a result of their personality or interaction style. These factors may therefore have profound effects in clinical studies, in particular pain-type studies, for example, a dentin hypersensitivity study, designed to evaluate the efficacy of various desensitising agents.

For example, a number of published studies evaluating desensitising toothpastes have demonstrated improvement in symptoms ranging from 30 to 80 % reduction in sensitivity when comparing test toothpastes to other toothpastes and placebo controls (Clark and Troullos 1990). The results from these studies are however somewhat conflicting and difficult to interpret, due in part to different methodologies and patient selection criteria. One of the main inherent problems in conducting clinical studies designed to assess the efficacy of desensitising products is the interference of placebo and/or Hawthorne effects that may introduce a degree of bias into the study (Gillam 1997, 2011; Addy et al. 2007). Several investigators have suggested that the utilisation of a double-blind placebo-controlled study is one possible way of resolving this particular bias, although such effects cannot be completely eliminated (Jeffcoat 1993; Holland et al. 1997; ADA Acceptance Program Guidelines 2012). For example, several investigators have reported that this effect can be as high as 40 % (Curro et al. 2000; West et al. 1997). Other investigators have also alluded to this effect in their published studies (Gillam et al. 1996, 1997a; Pearce et al. 1994; Chesters et al. 1992), but to what extent the placebo effect complicates the interpretation of the results of the study is difficult to predict. It should however be noted that according to Curro et al. (2000) the placebo effect observed in dentin hypersensitivity studies is not too dissimilar to those reported in other medical and dental therapeutic studies. For example, a review of 15 post-operative pain studies by Beecher (1955) cited by Curro et al. (2000) concluded that on average symptoms were satisfactorily relieved by the placebo medication in 35 % of the patients (the placebo response range of 15–58 %). According to Hróbjartsson and Gøtzsche (2001) in a systematic review detailing 27 trials involving the treatment of pain, the placebo had a beneficial effect, as indicated by a reduction in the intensity of pain of 6.5 mm on a 100-mm visual-analogue scale. If the magnitude of the placebo effect is reproduced in a clinical study, this may well confound any effects of efficacy of the active product. These and other confounding factors, for example, a random variation in patient symptoms over time (regression to the mean/mode, conditioning effects during the study, small sample size) affecting dentin hypersensitivity studies may also be complicated by the lack of universally acceptable positive and negative controls used in equivalence and superiority studies (Gillam 2011). A further problem that may confound determining the efficacy of these desensitising products is that the clinical efficacy of these products may be at the lower end of the therapeutic range (Addy et al. 2007). Curro et al. (2000) also suggested that subjects with chronic conditions such as dentin hypersensitivity typically have episodic or fluctuating symptoms and any potential change in these symptoms over time in a clinical study may be one of improvement (the so-called expectancy effect). A patient's expectancy of improvement may therefore influence outcomes as much as some active interventions, and this effect may be greater for novel interventions and for procedures (Oken 2008). It may therefore be suggested that the clinical study duration should be of a suitable duration (e.g. at least 6 weeks) as to minimise any 'placebo effects'.

It is important however to acknowledge that the amount of time required for a particular desensitising agent to achieve clinical effectiveness may be affected by several factors, including (a) variations in the motivation of individual patients and their ability to apply the product as intended and (b) the nature of the test agents and their likely mode of action. These factors may therefore dictate the design, nature and duration of any proposed clinical study.

5.5 Restorative Approaches

There are a number of restorative approaches for the treatment of DH that are provided for patients with localised moderate to severe DH which require immediate palliative alleviation (Orchardson and Gillam 2006). As indicated in Chap. 6, these desensitising agents may be classified on the basis of (1) whether products do not polymerise (varnishes/precipitants/primers containing HEMA), (2) whether they undergo setting or polymerisation reactions (conventional glass ionomer cements, or resin-reinforced glass [ionomers/compomers; adhesive resin primers; adhesive resin bonding systems), (3) the use of mouthguards, (4) iontophoresis combined with fluoride pastes or solutions and (5) lasers (Pashley 2000). Examples of these products are resins, varnishes, primers, dentine bonding agents and glass ionomer cements which contain fluoride, aluminium, potassium or ferric oxalates; silica or calcium-containing materials; and protein precipitants to decrease dentin permeability or block the fluid movement through dentin (Tables 5.3 and 5.4). Other miscellaneous treatment approaches have also been recommended, for example, occlusal adjustment associated with cervical abfraction lesion (Coleman et al. 2003), crown restorations, root coverage surgery, pulp extirpation, extraction (Ong and Strahan 1989), homoeopathic remedies (Plantago) (www.hpathy.com), propolis (Mahmound et al. 1999) and hypnosis (Starr et al. 1989; Eitner et al. 2010). It should however be acknowledged that some of these restorative procedures may also initiate post-operative sensitivity, for example, crown preparations, restorations, restorative materials, nonsurgical (scaling) and surgical procedures and sensitivity from bleaching or whitening procedures. One of the problems, however, when recommending or evaluating these restorative approaches for the treatment of dentin hypersensitivity is that dental professionals not only appear to be uncertain as to the most successful way in which to manage dentin hypersensitivity but also express a level of dissatisfaction with the various products and techniques available (Cunha-Cruz et al. 2010).

1. *Selected Non-polymerising Products*

   These products include varnishes/precipitants/primers containing HEMA.

   Historically varnishes and cavity liners such as Copalite have been recommended for the treatment of dentin hypersensitivity (Wycoff 1982), although most of these varnishes appear to provide inadequate insulation against thermal conduction under restorative materials (Voth et al. 1966). Varnishes such as copal varnishes (copal resin in an ether solution) were shown to be incompatible with the resin-based restorations due to their effect on the polymerisation process (Tjan and Chan 1987). As a result, a number of resin-compatible cavity varnishes, for example, Univar/Uniseal/Microjoin (Sci Pharm Duarte, Ca, USA) were introduced and evaluated on their ability to block dentin tubules (Tjan and Chan 1987; Tjan et al. 1987). Fluoride varnishes such as Duraphat® (Colgate Oral Pharmaceuticals), Dentinbloc (Colgate Oral Pharmaceuticals), Bifluorid 12 (VOCO GmbH), Isodan® (Septodont), Shellac F Cervitec® or Fluor Protector (Ivoclar Vivadent) have also been previously evaluated for the treatment of dentin hypersensitivity (Collaert et al. 1991; Thrash et al. 1992; Kielbassa et al. 1997; Gaffar 1999; Morris et al. 1999;

Table 5.3 Selected dentin desensitising solutions and products tested in clinical trials

Type, chemical/ concentration	Product and clinical support
Fluorides	
Sodium fluoride, stannous fluoride, hydrogen fluoride	Dentinbloc, Colgate Oral Pharmaceuticals, Canton MA, USA (Thrash et al. 1992; Morris et al. 1999)
Potassium nitrate	
1–15 % solutions	Hodash (1974)
5, 10 % in gel	Frechosa et al. (2003)
Oxalate	
3 % potassium oxalate	Protect, Sunstar Butler, Chicago, IL, USA Camps and Pashley (2003)
3 % potassium oxalate	Oxa-gel, Art-dent Ltda, Araraquara, SP, Brazil Pillon et al. (2004)
6.8 % ferric oxalate	Sensodyne Sealant, GSK, Jersey City NJ, USA Gillam et al. (2004)
Calcium phosphates	
1.5M calcium chloride + 1.0M potassium oxalate	Geiger et al. (2003)
D/Sense 2 (Centrix Direct)	Kolker et al. (2002) (in vitro)
Quell Desensitizer (Pentron Clinical Technologies)	

From Orchardson and Gillam (2006), Pashley et al. (2008) modified

Table 5.4 Selected professionally applied dentin desensitisers tested in clinical trials

Type	Product and clinical support
Fluoride varnish	Duraphat, Colgate Oral Pharmaceuticals, Canton, MA, USA (Gaffar 1999; Corona et al. 2003)
	Fluoline, PD Dental, Altenwalde, Germany (Duran and Sengun 2004)
	Duraflor (Pharmascience) (Merika et al. 2006)
	Fluor Protector (Ivoclar Vivadent)/AllSolutions Fluoride Varnish (Dentsply) (Ritter et al. 2006)
Oxalic acid + resin	MS Coat, Sun Medical Co, Shiga, Japan (Prati et al. 2001)
	Pain-Free, Parkell Co, Farmingdale, NY, USA (Morris et al. 1999)
Sealants, primers	Seal and Protect, Dentsply, Konstanz, Germany (Baysan and Lynch 2003; Aranha et al. 2009)
	Dentin Protector, Vivadent, Germany (Schwarz et al. 2002)
	Gluma Desensitizer, Heraeus Kulzer, Dormagen, Germany (Duran and Sengun 2004; Dondi dall' Orologio and Malferrari 1993, Dondi dall' Orologio et al. 1999, 2002; Polderman and Frencken 2007; Aranha et al. 2009; Mehmood et al. 2011)
	Gluma Alternate, Heraeus Kulzer, Wehrheim, Germany (Dondi dall'Orologio et al. 1999)
	Health-Dent Desensitizer, Healthdent Inc, Oswego, NY, USA (Duran and Sengun 2004; Dondi dall'Orologio et al. 1999)
	Hemaseal and Cide (Germiphene)/HurriSeal Dentin Desensitizer (Beutlich Pharm.) (Kolker et al. 2002)
	One-Step (Bisco, USA) (Kakaboura et al. 2005)
	Prime and Bond 2.1, Dentsply Caulk, Milford, DE, USA (Swift et al. 2001)
	Scotchbond (Single Bond), 3M Dental Products, St Paul, MN, USA (Duran and Sengun 2004; Prati et al. 2001; Ferrari et al. 1999)
Etch + primer	Scotchbond, 3M Dental Products, St Paul, MN, USA (Ferrari et al. 1999)
	Systemp.desensitizer, Ivoclar Vivadent, Schaan, Liechtenstein (Stewardson et al. 2004)
Etch + primer + adhesive	Scotchbond Multi-Purpose Adhesive, 3M Dental Products, St Paul, MN, USA (Dondi dall'Orologio et al. 1999)
Primer + adhesive	SE Bond, Kuraray, Okayama, Japan (Duran and Sengun 2004)
Glass ionomer cements	Resin-modified glass ionomer liner (Vitrebond 3M ESPE) (Hansen 1992; Tantbirojn et al. 2006)
	Fuji VII (GC) (Polderman et al. 2007)

From Orchardson and Gillam (2006), Pashley et al. (2008) modified

Panduric et al. 2001; Merika et al. 2006; Ritter et al. 2006; Hoang-Dao et al. 2009; Bhandary and Hegde 2012). According to Ritter et al. (2006), the topical application of fluoride varnishes was thought to create a barrier by the precipitation of CaF_2 onto the exposed dentin surface which, in turn may occlude the dentin tubules thereby reducing dentin permeability and, as a consequence, DH. From a practical viewpoint, the application of a fluoride varnish may be useful in identifying whether a patient has DH during the diagnosis examination in order to rule out any other dental cause. The application of fluoride varnishes may also be incorporated in a stepwise management programme where non-invasive procedures are undertaken, and depending on whether the problem has been resolved or not, the clinician may either proceed to provide additional applications of the varnish or opt to provide a more invasive procedure (Orchardson and Gillam 2006). Other treatment approaches include the application of Hema-containing primers, for example, Gluma (5 % glutaraldehyde primer and 35 % hydroxyethyl methacrylate), calcium hydroxide and oxalate varnishes (Pashley 2000; Orchardson and Gillam 2006) (Tables 5.3 and 5.4). The efficacy of Hema-containing primers in treating DH has been evaluated in a number of clinical studies. For example, Felton et al. (1991) applied the primer to the facial surfaces of crown preparations in 20 patients and reported that in response to air, tactile and osmotic stimuli, DH was significantly reduced after 14 days compared to the control group. Other investigators (Dondi dall' Orologio and Malferrari 1993, Dondi dall' Orologio et al. 1999, 2002; Duran and Sengun 2004) reported similar successful results when using the primer on exposed dentin. However a study by de Assis et al. (2006) in periodontal patients with hypersensitive teeth failed to demonstrate any efficacy with Gluma Desensitizer® compared to the control group. A more recent study by Mehmood et al. (2011) compared Gluma Desensitizer® with Duraphat® in 196 patients with non-carious cervical lesions. They conclude that Gluma Desensitizer® significantly reduced DH compared to the Duraphat® varnish. A 6-month study by Aranha et al. (2009) evaluated Gluma Desensitizer® with four other products or therapies (Seal and Protect, OXA GEL, fluoride and low-intensity laser treatment). They concluded that although both Gluma Desensitizer® and Seal and Protect had an immediate effect in reducing DH, all therapies demonstrated lower sensitivity scores at the 6-month evaluation point. The proposed mechanism of blocking the tubules with HEMA-containing primers may be a result of the glutaraldehyde component reacting with the albumin within the dentin fluid by protein precipitation; this in turn may reduce the outward fluid flow and as a consequence reduce DH (Pashley 2000).

The application of oxalate-containing solutions has also been evaluated for treating DH (Muzzin and Johnson 1989; Salvato et al. 1990; Kerns et al. 1991; Morris et al. 1999; Gillam et al. 1997, 2004; Pashley et al. 2001; Camps and Pashley 2003; Tay et al. 2003; Pillon et al. 2004; Pamir et al. 2007) although according to Pashley (2000) and Orchardson and Gillam (2000), the clinical evidence is somewhat inconclusive. In this context it is of interest that despite this reservation on the efficacy of these products, 40 % of practising dentists in the USA reported using oxalate preparations in order to treat DH (Cunha-Cruz et al. 2010). A systematic review by Cunha-Cruz et al. (2011) concluded that many of the oxalate products that were included for evaluation in the review were no better than the placebo controls with the possible exception of a 3 % monohydrogen monopotassium oxalate solution. These investigators concluded that the current evidence did not support recommending using oxalates for the treatment of DH. The mechanism by which oxalate products block the dentin tubules has been demonstrated by a number of investigators (Greenhill and Pashley 1981; Gillam et al. 2001; Yiu et al. 2005). According to Yiu et al. (2005) following the application of the oxalate solution on the depletion of calcium ions from the surface dentin forces the oxalate ions to diffuse further down into the dentin tubule and react to form insoluble calcium oxalate crystals. This reaction results in a subsurface tubular occlusion which will reduce fluid flow (dentin permeability) within the dentin tubules.

According to Pashley (2000), the use of calcium hydroxide paste has been applied for the treatment of DH. For example, Green et al. (1997) applied a 5-min treatment of calcium hydroxide on hypersensitive root surfaces and reported that in response to thermal and mechanical stimuli, DH was reduced for the duration of the 3-month study. Wolfart et al. (2004) also compared a calcium hydroxide solution with a glutaraldehyde-based dentin primer in 36 patients undergoing crown preparations and evaluated over a 30-month period. Although the investigators reported that a calcium hydroxide solution may be useful in treating DH, there were no reported differences between the two products. According to Ling and Gillam (1996) citing McFall (1986), calcium hydroxide blocks the dentin tubules by a deposition of calcium ions that bind to free protein radicals and increasing the remineralisation of the exposed dentin. It was claimed that the initial application was successful for 80–90 % of the time, but this effect rapidly diminished and frequent reapplication was required. Pashley et al. (1986) applied a calcium hydroxide paste to human dentin in vitro in order to determine its effects on dentin permeability. The results indicated that although the paste reduced dentin permeability in both smear layer and non-smear layer samples, calcium hydroxide provides little protection to an acid challenge. On the basis of these studies, it would appear that the use of calcium hydroxide on exposed root surfaces may be of limited value.

2. *Selected Products That Undergo Setting or Polymerisation Reactions*

These products include conventional glass ionomer cements, or resin-reinforced glass ionomers/compomers; adhesive resin primers; and adhesive resin bonding systems.

The use of conventional glass ionomer cements (GIC) or resin-reinforced glass ionomers/compomers has been recommended for a number of clinical conditions in the oral cavity, for example, as a liner in prepared cavities (Hansen 1992; Tantbirojn et al. 2006; Burrow et al. 2009), fissure sealing (Pardi et al. 2003), cementing orthodontic brackets (Charles 1998), treatment of dentin hypersensitivity (Wycoff 1982), non-carious cervical lesions (Francisconi et al. 2009) and a combined surgical/restorative intervention of gingival recession with associated non-carious cervical lesions (Santamaria et al. 2007). It should however be acknowledged that the term 'glass ionomer cement' is loosely applied in the published literature and therefore may be somewhat misleading as there are differences between the original GIC product and the various resin-modified and composite resin materials that have been developed over the last 20–30 years. From a clinical point of view, it is important to note that they may bind differently to the tooth surface depending on whether they are a conventional GIC or a resin-modified GIC (Tyas and Burrows 2004). According to Mount et al. (2009), with the conventional GIC or a resin-modified GIC, there is an ion exchange adhesion with the tooth surface via a polyacid interaction even though the initiation may be different (acid–base setting/acid–base setting plus photoinitiation). There is also a sustained fluoride release from the material as well as a subsequent fluoride recharging from the oral environment over time has also been demonstrated. With both the conventional and polyacid-modified composite resin systems there does not appear to be any particular benefit apart from a minimal benefit via a polyacid reaction of the polyacid-modified composite resin system (Mount et al. 2009). Several investigators have used various GIC products to treat DH, for example, Low (1981) reported a reduction in sensitivity following the placement of the material in cervical abrasion lesions. Polderman and Frencken (2007) also reported that a low-viscosity glass ionomer (Fuji VII) was more effective in treating DH than Gluma Desensitizer after 3 months and after 24 months.

The rationale of using adhesive restorative materials (dentin bonding agents, resins and adhesives) for the treatment of DH was based on the possibility of blocking the dentin tubules (Brännström et al. 1979; Pashley 1992b). Results from the initial studies using these materials indicated that there was an immediate and long-lasting effect in reducing DH except when the adhesive sheared off the dentin surface resulting in a return to the previous baseline values (Ling and Gillam 1996). According to Tyas and Burrows (2004), the mechanism by which these materials bond to the dentin is via a hybrid layer or resin-impregnated layer. Basically this is a micromechanical interlocking of resin around the collagen fibrils exposed by the demineralisation process during the pretreatment phase when placing the material onto the dentin surface. From a clinical viewpoint, these materials offer a challenge to the dental practitioner as they are very technique sensitive and require careful handling and manipulation. It is essential that the dental professional follow the instructions from the manufacturer very carefully when placing the material in the oral environment. Furthermore it is also important that the dental professional has an understanding of the characteristics associated with both conventional glass ionomer cements, or resin-reinforced glass ionomers/compomers, and adhesive restorative materials in order to maximise the usefulness of these materials in the oral environment.

According to Orchardson and Gillam (2006), the dental professional should be aware of the pragmatic nature of the published clinical studies of adhesive desensitising materials. For example, many of the reported studies are single-blind studies because true double-blind conditions are difficult to achieve. A further problem when analysing results from the published literature is that there has been a major change in the available products since the original introduction of dentin bonding agents, resins and adhesives. A selection of published studies that claim to relieve DH by blocking the dentin are presented in Table 5.4 (based on Orchardson and Gillam 2006 and Pashley et al. 2008 published reviews). A recent 6-month study by Veitz-Keenan et al. (2013) reported on the use of a potassium nitrate toothpaste, sealant (one-step self-etch dentin bonding agent [Clearfil S3 Bond, Kuraray, Okayama, Japan]/Clearfil Liner Bond 2 Protect Liner F, Kuraray) or restoration (dentin bonding agent [Clearfil S3 Bond]/flowable composite resin [Premise Flowable, Kerr]) for the treatment of hypersensitive non-carious cervical lesions. The results indicated that both the sealant and the restoration treatment proved equally effective for most participants in reducing dentin hypersensitivity in non-carious cervical lesions.

The application of both adhesive restorative materials (dentin, bonding agents, resins and adhesives) would therefore appear best suited to localised rather than generalised areas of dentin hypersensitivity and would appear to be ideal for using within the stepwise minimal intervention approach as suggested by Orchardson and Gillam (2006).

3. *Use of Mouthguards*

According to Haywood (2000) and Tredwin et al. (2006), tooth sensitivity is a common adverse reaction of external bleaching procedures. It has also been reported in the literature that patients who have a pre-existing history of DH or with gingival recession and associated DH may be more likely to experience DH during the bleaching process (Leonard et al. 2004). For patients with pre-existing dentin hypersensitivity, the use of a desensitising product, for example, 5 % potassium nitrate (toothpaste or in a bleaching tray), prior to bleaching the teeth may alleviate further discomfort during the bleaching phase of the treatment (Haywood et al. 2001, 2005). Other products such as amorphous calcium phosphate (ACP) have also been recommended for the prevention of DH/bleaching sensitivity either as a toothpaste or as a professionally applied product (Giniger et al. 2005). According to Haywood (2002), the incidence of DH/bleaching sensitivity ranges between 55 and 75 % of subjects undergoing bleaching procedures in randomised clinical trials.

Several investigators have suggested that bleaching sensitivity is mediated by a hydrodynamic mechanism (Croll 2003; Swift 2005; Markowitz 2010). Croll (2003) described a mechanism where oxygen bubbles from the carbamide or hydrogen peroxide form in the dentin tubules during the bleaching process and initiate dentin fluid movements that in turn may activate the intradental nerves. No evidence however has been advanced to support this interesting hypothesis although the hydrodynamic hypothesis does not appear to fully explain the mechanism of pain associated with the bleaching process.

4. *Iontophoresis Combined with Fluoride Pastes or Solutions*

Several investigators have recommended the use and application of fluoride with or without iontophoresis (Gangarosa and Park 1978; Brough et al. 1985; Gupta et al. 2010; Aparna et al. 2010) although the clinical efficacy of this technique has been questioned (Gillam and Newman 1990; Pashley 2000).

5. *Lasers*

The use of laser technology has been advocated by several investigators for the treatment of DH (Renton-Harper and Midda 1992; Kimura et al. 2000; Yilmaz et al. 2011a, b; Umberto et al. 2012). The evidence for the efficacy of this therapy is, however, somewhat equivocal (West 2007; He et al. 2011) (see Chap. 6). According to Kimura et al. (2000), the rationale and mechanism of how laser therapy is effective in treating DH is inadequately explained. A number of investigators have proposed that lasers may work either through a process which involves the coagulation and precipitation of plasma proteins in the dentin fluid (Pashley 2000) or by the effect of the emitted thermal energy from the laser altering intradental nerve activity (Orchardson et al. 1997, 1998). McCarthy et al. (1997) however reported that both Nd:YAG and Er:YAG lasers caused alteration of the dentin surface either by melting and re-solidification of the dentin with partially blocked tubules (Nd:YAG) or by ablation of the dentin surface leaving craters and open tubules (in the dentin discs) or blocked tubules (on the root surface) (Er:YAG), but neither lasers produced a smooth glazed impermeable surface. There are a number of different laser systems that have been recommended by investigators for the treatment of DH, for example, neodymium-doped yttrium, aluminium and garnet (Nd:YAG); erbium and chromium to yttrium, scandium and gallium (Er,Cr:YSG); erbium and chromium doped to yttrium, scandium, gallium and garnet (Er,Cr:YSGG); carbon dioxide (CO_2); and diode lasers. Several investigators have also combined various lasers with fluoride varnishes and potassium nitrate gels in order to treat DH, for example, GaAlAs (BDP 600), Co_2, Er:YAG or Nd:YAG lasers and a sodium fluoride gel or varnish (Corona et al. 2003; Ipci et al. 2009); Kara and Orbak 2009 or a 810 nm diode laser and a 10 % potassium nitrate bioadhesive gel (Sicilia et al. 2009). These investigators reported positive results with the combined application of a laser and fluoride gel or varnish; however these studies had relatively small numbers of subjects per group, and therefore further well-controlled studies are required to determine whether there would be an added benefit to the patient. Several investigators have recently undertaken reviews (systematic review/meta-analysis) on the efficacy of in-office treatments or laser therapy for the treatment of DH (Lin et al. 2013; Sgolastra et al. 2013). These investigators reported that laser therapy was efficacious in reducing DH compared to a placebo control. Lin et al. (2013) however indicated that there were no significant differences between the different treatment modalities. Although laser therapy appears to be an area of interest from a research viewpoint, there appears to be limited use of lasers in dental practice when treating DH (Cunha-Cruz et al. 2010).

6. *Other Miscellaneous Treatment*

   A large number of anecdotal reports support alternative approaches for treating DH. Although these reports are not truly evidence based, they may be applied to some clinical situations. For example, periodontal surgery involving coronally positioned flaps reportedly eliminates dentin hypersensitivity in exposed root dentin (See Sect. 5.5). If DH is associated with an abfraction lesion, occlusal adjustment may also be effective (Coleman et al. 2003). Other miscellaneous procedures for the treatment of DH were reported, for example, burnishing exposed root surfaces (Ling and Gillam 1996; Pashley 2000), crown restorations, pulp extirpation, extraction (Ong and Strahan 1989) and hypnosis (Starr et al. 1989; Eitner et al. 2010).

5.5.1 Post-operative Sensitivity from Restorative Approaches

A review of the published literature would indicate that post-operative sensitivity from restorative treatment is a commonly reported feature in dental practice. One of the problems in determining the actual prevalence of the problem however, was that some of the published studies were mainly anecdotal reports in nature and as such were prone to reporting bias when claiming the elimination of post-operative sensitivity with products which use dental adhesive liners. According to Haywood (2002), there are a number of factors associated with the placement of restorations in vivo, for example, certain amalgam materials have been shown to cause post-operative sensitivity (restorative sensitivity) of up to 48 h due to shrinkage of the material rather than the predicted expansion during setting. Other factors include the contamination of composites during placement or improper etching of the tooth during tooth preparation which may result in micro-leakage; improper technique when drying the tooth or incorrect preparation of materials such as glass ionomer or zinc phosphate cements may also be problematic. The techniques involved in cavity preparation may also affect the integrity of the pulp initiating an inflammatory response and subsequent pain as well as thermal changes due to the choice of the restorative material used to restore the tooth. Galvanic reactions due to dissimilar metals have also been reported to cause post-operative pain (Haywood 2002). Porto (2012) has also suggested that there are a number of factors that may initiate post-operative sensitivity with the placement of direct resin composite restorations (Table 5.5). As previously indicated tooth sensitivity has been reported to be associated with bleaching procedures (Haywood 2000; Tredwin et al. 2006), and a number of treatment strategies have been recommend as indicated above.

Table 5.5 Possible causes of pre- and post-operative sensitivity from direct resin composites

Preoperative causes	Operative causes	Post-operative causes
Cracks and fractures	Abusive dental structure wear by instruments	Restorative finishing and polishing
Cervical dentin exposure	Dehydration of the dentin	Occlusal interference
Condition of the pulp	Incomplete caries removal	Cervical dentin exposure
	Negligence in protecting the dentin–pulp complex Increase in cavity depth Inadequate isolation of the operative field Failure in dental tissue hybridisation Handling the restorative material Polymerisation shrinkage (contraction stress). Incomplete resin composite polymerisation Flow characteristics of composites	

From Porto (2012)

According to Berkowitz et al. (2009), post-operative sensitivity following the placement of posterior resin-based composites is a common concern in general dental practice although the evidence for this statement is limited.

Several investigators have however suggested that one method of relieving post-operative sensitivity is by the adjunctive use of oxalate desensitisers on acid-etched dentin prior to adhesive application (Pashley et al. 2001; Tay et al. 2003). Yiu et al. (2005) however urged caution on the use of oxalate desensitisers under certain conditions, in particular with acidic, fluoride-containing total-etch adhesives due to their incompatibility problems.

According to Gillam and Orchardson (2006), DH is a common occurrence following periodontal surgery and root scaling/debridement although with well-controlled oral hygiene procedures, this problem appears to resolve over time (Tammaro et al. 2000). Several investigators have also reported that the prevalence of DH is in the region of 9–27 % before and 54–55 % following periodontal therapy (von Troil et al. 2002; Lin and Gillam 2012). The reported intensity from DH increased up to 4 weeks following these procedures, after which the recorded values returned back to the original baseline scores (Gillam and Orchardson 2006). A number of studies have also indicated that a relatively small number of patients (1.3–7 %) complain of severe DH following treatment of infrabony defects with an enamel matrix derivative (Zetterstrom et al. 1997; Heard et al. 2000; Froum et al. 2004). It is important to note that for most patients post-operative sensitivity is of a transient nature and may be adequately managed by the clinician using the recommended materials and procedures outlined in Chaps. 5 and 6. If the post-operative sensitivity has not resolved within 6 weeks, it is recommended that further investigations be undertaken to determine the cause of the problem and treat accordingly.

5.6 Periodontal Surgical Techniques

According to Gillam and Orchardson (2006), periodontal grafts and guided tissue regeneration (GTR) procedures have been described in the published literature for the treatment of gingival recession with DH. These procedures generally have predictable outcomes and may therefore be the treatment of choice for patients since this may provide a good aesthetic as well as palliative solution to their clinical problem (Drisko 2002). Both aesthetics and pain from DH have been reported as the main concerns of patients when seeking treatment (Pagliaro et al. 2003; Zaher et al. 2005). Previously one of the problems when evaluating the efficacy of the root coverage procedures and associated DH was that there was only limited evidence-based data available on the actual extent of the problem of DH before and following the procedure(s) (Gillam and Orchardson 2006). Furthermore the results from the published clinical studies generally evaluated the success or failure of specific technique and procedures with DH as an unpleasant side effect from the surgical procedure rather than specifically evaluate patients with exposed root dentin with associated DH. For example, Al-Hamdan et al. (2003) in a meta-analysis review while acknowledging that the indications for initiating root coverage procedures included DH reported that the 40 papers included in the review provided no evidence to either determine the prevalence or extent of the problem in patients with gingival recession. This observation was also substantiated by Pagliaro et al. (2003) who reported that out of the 90 accepted papers included in the review, DH was generally identified as being either present or absent in 19 papers (21.1 %) and only nine articles (10 %) recorded any pre- and post-treatment data, with only two of these studies quantifying DH on a recognised 10-point pain scale.

Several investigators have suggested that if the root coverage of the gingival defect cannot be predictably treated by conventional surgical root coverage procedures, then the remaining exposed cervical dentin could be treated with a more invasive restorative material (Tugnait and Clerehugh 2001; Drisko 2002). This may be as a result of either patient-related factors or an extensive loss of interdental gingival and bone tissue as a result of periodontal disease. Open gingival embrasures, also called 'black triangles', may be produced interfering with the aesthetics of the smile (Sharma and Park 2010). A relatively simple nonsurgical approach to this problem was proposed by Greene (1998) who suggested the construction of a flexible gingival mask of silicone using a simple two-stage impression technique. Localised recession defects may also be addressed by using a partial laminate porcelain veneer technique (Capa 2007). Zalkind and Hochman (1997) also recommended the use of tooth-coloured composite as a minimally invasive adhesive restoration. The latter restorative technique may also resolve associated carious lesions and alleviate pain symptoms from DH (Zalkind and Hochman 1997). Restoration of a non-carious/carious cervical lesion with glass ionomer cements may also have the added advantage of fluoride release over a prolonged period of time (Özgünaltay and Önen 2002). A combined surgical and restorative approach has been described by Santamaria et al. (2007) in three case reports of patients with Miller's Class I gingival margin defect with associated non-carious cervical lesions. These authors recommended a combined surgical/restorative approach using a coronally advanced flap procedure with/without a connective tissue graft together with a resin-modified glass ionomer restoration when dealing with this particular problem. However as these investigators acknowledged, further longitudinal randomised clinical trials are required to support this combined approach to correcting gingival recession defects and associated non-carious cervical lesions. If the non-carious cervical lesion is below the cementum–enamel junction, this may cause problems when adapting the gingival flap to the root surface, and modification of the root surface to eliminate the concavity of the lesion may require reshaping of the root surface using diamond finishing burs (Santamaria et al. 2007). It is however imperative that clinicians should avoid placing subgingival restorations whenever possible in order to prevent plaque retention as well as maintaining the biological width when placing crowns (Drisko 2002).

Several investigators have reported that there is an increase in DH following scaling and periodontal surgery although this effect may be transient in nature (von Troil et al. 2002; Gillam and Orchardson 2006). One possible explanation for this observation is that periodontal procedures such as scaling may initially uncover the dentin tubules (a created smear layer) exposing them to the oral environment thus causing patients transient pain when eating or drinking in the days following the procedures. It is evident however that a smear layer may be covering the dentinal tubules since the cementum would have been removed in order for the root dentine to be exposed (Pashley 1984). Natural occlusion may also occur due to the precipitation of salivary constituents onto the tooth surface (Kerns et al. 1991; Kawasaki et al. 2001). Several investigators have speculated that scaling and root planing procedures may remove 20–50 μm of cementum thus exposing the dentinal tubules to external stimuli (Nishida et al. 1976; Wallace and Bissada 1990). It has also been suggested that bacterial invasion of exposed cementum associated with periodontal disease occurs after the cementum has been altered by physiological, bacterial or environmental factors (Love and Jenkinson 2002). The implications on the integrity of the pulp as a result of bacterial invasion of the dentin tubules may therefore depend on whether the pulpo-dentin defences are able to withstand this insult. According to Love and Jenkinson (2002), it is likely that the dentin fluid components including albumin, fibrinogen and IgG are involved in host defence by interacting directly with bacteria and metabolites and by reducing the permeability of dentin. It has been speculated that any bacterial invasion of the dentin tubules would have a greater impact on outward fluid flow than with inward diffusion of noxious substances due to changes in the tubular radius rather than with diffusion characteristics of bulk fluid movements per se (Pashley 1992a, b). This speculation was however based on in vitro observations and does not appear to have been substantiated in clinical practice. Several investigators have recommended the use of a topical fluoride or a desensitising polishing paste application with a view to alleviate patient discomfort following scaling and root planing procedures (Paine et al. 1998; Hamlin et al. 2009; Schiff et al. 2009a, b; Milleman et al. 2012; Li et al. 2013; Neuhaus et al. 2013). Oxalate solutions have also been advocated for post-operative hypersensitivity, for example, Wang et al. (1993) applied a 6 % ferric oxalate solution during periodontal surgery and Pillon et al. (2004) applied a 3 % potassium oxalate application following subgingival scaling and root planing. Both investigators reported a reduction in post-operative hypersensitivity following application of the oxalate solutions.

From a treatment and management perspective, a number of classifications have been previously proposed in the published literature in order to facilitate both a diagnosis and a template for the correction of gingival margin defects. Currently the classification used in root coverage procedures is the Miller classification system ([I–IV] (Miller 1985). An example of Miller's Class I defect may be seen in Fig. 5.3. The advantage of this classification is the ability to correlate treatment prognosis/outcome and anatomical features, whereas previous classification systems used either anatomical features or treatment prognosis only. A number of materials and techniques have been reported in the literature, and these include guided tissue regeneration (GTR), coronally advanced flap and Emdogain (CAF + EMD), connective tissue graft (CTG) and free gingival graft (acellular dermal matrix allograft/ Mucograft ADM) (Table 5.6, Fig. 5.4a, b). A recent systemic review by Douglas de Oliveira et al. (2013), however, suggested that currently there is insufficient scientific evidence to

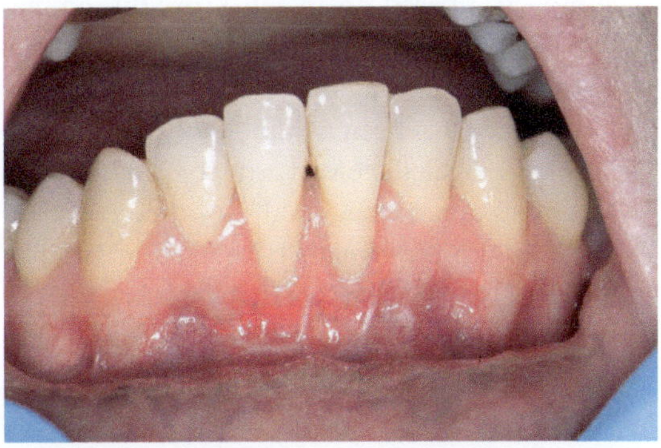

Fig. 5.3 Miller Class I defect of a patient complaining of DH following completion of the orthodontic treatment. The patient was referred in order to provide root coverage of the lower central incisors (Acknowledgement KN Al Shayeb)

Table 5.6 Periodontal flap surgery/periodontal plastic surgical techniques

Material/technique	Proposed mode of action
Guided tissue regeneration (GTR)	Root coverage of the exposed dentin by connective tissue flaps, guided tissue regeneration (GTR) with or without enamel matrix derivatives or acellular dermal matrix/Mucograft (e.g., Saadoun 2008, Sanz et al. 2009, Dominiak et al. 2012). In vitro and clinical evidence for these products and procedures has been demonstrated, and there is some histological evidence that these products have the potential to regenerate bone. For example, selective repopulation of a root surface by periodontal ligament cells forming new connective tissue attachment between the root surface and alveolar bone may be achieved using GTR procedures. Connective tissue grafts with or without enamel matrix derivatives or acellular dermal matrix/Mucograft may also result in increased keratinisation of the gingiva (Alghamdi et al. 2009). Successful coverage of the root surface would therefore provide a physical barrier that may in turn decrease DH
Coronally advanced flap and Emdogain (CAF + EMD)	
Connective tissue graft (CTG)	
Free gingival graft (acellular dermal matrix allograft/ Mucograft ADM)	

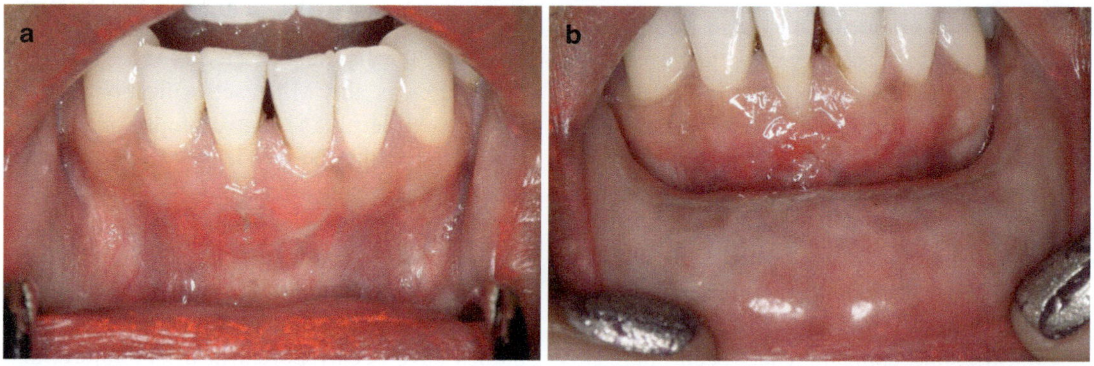

Fig. 5.4 (**a**) Clinical photograph of a Miller Class III with fenestration (Pre-operative). Patient was complaining of gingival sensitivity associated with the mandibular lower left central incisor (Acknowledgement KN Al Shayeb). (**b**) Clinical photograph of the Miller Class III defect 1 week post op

conclude that surgical root coverage procedures predictably reduce DH.

Conclusions

The hydrodynamic theory promotes two basic approaches based on in vitro, in situ, animal and human studies for treating DH, namely, blocking dentin tubules and nerve desensitising. There have been a number of reviews that have investigated the vast array of products and treatment approaches (both in-office or OTC) that dental professionals have used in order to treat DH, and it is evident that there is no widespread agreement as to which is the best material or procedure to treat DH (Gillam 1992; Orchardson and Gillam 2006; Cunha-Cruz et al. 2010; Lin et al. 2013). One of the problems however in evaluating the effectiveness of desensitising products is the variability in the methodology, sample size and duration used in the published clinical trials. Other factors that may influence the efficacy of the product under test in clinical studies include the impact of placebo and non-placebo effects, the random variation in patient symptoms over time (regression to the mean/mode) and the relationship between the subject and the examiner. It is also evident that patients may experience post-operative sensitivity from the various procedures in the dental office, for example, from restorative procedures, restorations, crowns, bleaching of the teeth and nonsurgical and surgical procedures. Although these effects may be of a transient nature, they may cause undue distress to the patient and their quality of life which may in turn necessitate further treatment. This may include simple reassurance and monitoring or further investigation and treatment of the particular problem. It is essential that the patient is monitored within a practical management programme, and in most situations a stepwise approach (minimally invasive) including preventive measures may be incorporated (see Chap. 6). The use of this stepwise approach as proposed by Orchardson and Gillam (2006) may enable the dental professional to use a combination of products, restorative approaches and treatment philosophies in order to successfully treat DH.

References

ADA Acceptance Program Guidelines (2012) Products for the treatment of dentinal hypersensitivity. American Dental Association, Council for Scientific Affairs, April 2012, Chicago, IL, USA. www.ada.org/sections/scienceAndResearch/pdfs/Products. Accessed Jan 2014

Addy M, Dowell P (1983) Dentine and hypersensitivity-a review. Clinical and in vitro evaluation of treatment agents. J Clin Periodontol 10:351–366

Addy M, Mostafa P, Newcombe R (1987) Dentine hypersensitivity. A comparison of five toothpastes used during a 6-week treatment period. BDJ 163:45–50

Addy M, Loyn T, Adams D (1991) Dentine hypersensitivity – effects of some proprietary mouthwashes on the dentine smear layer. A SEM Study J Dent 19:148–152

Addy M, West NX, Barlow A, Smith S (2007) Dentine hypersensitivity: is there both stimulus and placebo responses in clinical trials? Int J Dent Hygiene 5:53–59

Ajcharanukul O, Kraivaphan P, Wanachantararak S, Vongsavan N, Matthews B (2007) Effects of potassium ions on dentine sensitivity in man. Arch Oral Biol 52:632–639

Ajcharanukul O, Chidchuangchai W, Charoenlarp P, Vongsavan N, Matthews B (2011) Sensory transduction in human teeth with inflamed pulps. J Dent Res 90(5):678–682

Ajcharanukul O, Wanachantararak S, Vongsavan N, Matthews B (2012) Repeated hydrostatic pressure stimulation of dentin in man. In: Presentation (abstract no. 3249), 90th general session and exhibition of the IADR Iguaçu Falls, Brazil, 20–23 June

Alghamdi H, Babay N, Sukumaran A (2009) Surgical management of gingival recession: a clinical update. Saudi Dent J 21(2):83–94

Al-Hamdan K, Eber R, Sarment D, Kowalski C, Wang H-L (2003) Guided tissue regeneration-based root coverage: meta-analysis. J Periodontol 74:1520–1533

Anderson DJ (1968) The pulp as a sensory organ. In: Finn SB (ed) Biology of the dental pulp organ. University of Alabama Press, Birmingham, pp 273–280

Anderson DJ (1972) Human and animal studies on sensory mechanisms in teeth. J Dent Res 22:33–38

Anderson DJ, Naylor MN (1962a) Chemical excitants of pain in human dentine. Arch Oral Biol 7:413–415

Anderson DJ, Ronning GA (1962b) Osmotic excitants of pain in human dentine. Arch Oral Biol 7:513–523

Anderson DJ, Curwen MP, Howard LV (1958) The sensitivity of human dentin. J Dent Res 37:669–677

Aranha ACC, Pimenta LAF, Marchi GM (2009) Clinical evaluation of desensitizing treatments for cervical dentin hypersensitivity. Braz Oral Res 23(3):333–339

Aparna S, Setty S, Thakur S (2010) Comparative efficacy of two treatment modalities for dentinal hypersensitivity: a clinical trial. Indian J Dent Res 21(4):544–548. doi:10.4103/0970-9290.74213

Ayad F, Ayad N, Delgado E, Zhang YP, DeVizio W, Cummins D, Mateo LR (2009) Comparing the efficacy in providing instant relief of dentin hypersensitivity of a new toothpaste containing 8.0% arginine, calcium carbonate, and 1450 ppm fluoride to a benchmark, desensitizing toothpaste containing 2% potassium ion and 1450ppm fluoride, and to a control toothpaste with 1450ppm fluoride. A three-day clinical study in Mississauga, Canada. J Clin Dent 20:115–122

Azarpazhooh A, Limeback H (2008) Clinical efficacy of casein derivatives: a systematic review of the literature. J Am Dent Assoc 139(7):915–924

Baysan A, Lynch E (2003) Treatment of cervical sensitivity with a root sealant. Am J Dent 16(2):135–138

Beecher HK (1955) The powerful placebo. J Am Med Assoc 159:1602–1606

Berkowitz GS, Horowitz AJ, Fredrick A, Curro FA, Craig RG et al (2009) Postoperative hypersensitivity in class I resin-based composite restorations in general practice: interim results. Compend Contin Educ Dent 30(6):356–363

Bhandary S, Hedge MN (2012) A clinical comparison of in office management of dentin hypersensitivity in a short term treatment period. IJBAR 03(03):69–174. ijbar.ssjournals.com/index.php/journal/article/download/114/638

Blitzer B (1967) A consideration of the possible causes of dental hyper- sensitivity: treatment by a strontium-ion dentifrice. Periodontics 5:318–321

Brännström M (1963) A hydrodynamic mechanism in the transmission of pain-produced stimuli through the dentine. In: Anderson DJ (ed) Sensory mechanisms in dentine. Pergamon, Oxford, pp 73–79

Brännström M, Johnson G, Nordenvall K-J (1979) Transmission and control of dentinal pain: resin impregnation for the desensitization of dentin. JADA 99:612–618

Brauer DS, Karpukhina N, O'Donnell MD, Law RV, Hill RG (2010) Fluoride-containing bioactive glasses: effect of glass design and structure on degradation, pH and apatite formation in simulated body fluid. Acta Biomater 6:3275–3282

Brough KM, Anderson DM, Love J, Overman PR (1985) The effectiveness of iontophoresis in reducing dentin hypersensitivity. J Am Dent Assoc 111(5):761–765

Burrow MF, Banomyong D, Harnirattisai C, Messer HH (2009) Effect of glass-ionomer cement lining on

postoperative sensitivity in occlusal cavities restored with resin composite–a randomized clinical trial. Oper Dent 34(6):648–655
Burwell A (2006) Tubule occlusion of a Novamin-containing dentifrice compared to Recaldent-containing dentifrice – a Remin/Demin study in vitro. Novamin research reports
Burwell AK, Litkowski LJ, Greenspan DC (2009) Calcium sodium phosphosilicate (NovaMin): remineralization potential. Adv Dent Res 21(1):35–39
Camps J, Pashley D (2003) In vivo sensitivity of human root dentin to air blast and scratching. J Periodontol 74:1589–1594
Capa N (2007) Alternative treatment approach to gingival recession: gingival-colored partial porcelain veneer: a clinical report. J Prosthet Dent 98:82–84
Charig AJ, Chapin CA, Major EE, Thong S et al (2009) Mechanism of action of a desensitizing fluoride toothpaste delivering calcium and phosphate ingredients in the treatment of dental hypersensitivity. Part I: in vitro Sem, Edx, profilometry, and dentin permeability studies. Compendium 30(8). Online access only
Charles C (1998) Bonding orthodontic brackets with glass-ionomer cement. Biomaterials 19(6):589–591
Cherng AM, Chow LC, Takagi S (2004) Reduction in dentin permeability using mildly supersaturated calcium phosphate solutions. Arch Oral Biol 49(2):91–98
Chesters R, Kaufman HW, Wolff MS, Huntington E, Kleinberg I (1992) Use of multiple sensitivity measurements and logit statistical analysis to assess the effectiveness of a potassium citrate-containing dentifrice in reducing dentinal hypersensitivity. J Clin Periodontol 19:256–261
Clark GE, Troullos ES (1990) Designing hypersensitivity clinical studies. Dent Clin North Am 34:531–544
Cohen S (1961) Efficacy of a dentifrice containing potassium. J Periodontol 32:49–53, 56
Coleman TA, Grippo JO, Kinderknecht KE (2003) Cervical dentin hyper-sensitivity. Part III: resolution following occlusal equilibration. Quintessence Int 34:427–434
Collaert B, De Bruyn H, Söderholm G, Brattthall GT (1991) Evaluation of a fluoride varnish for dentine sensitivity treatment. J Dent Res 70:83 (Abstr no 102)
Corona SAM, Nascimento NT, Catirse ABE, Lizarelli RFZ et al (2003) Clinical evaluation of low-level laser therapy and fluoride varnish for treating cervical dentinal hypersensitivity. J Oral Rehabil 30:1183–1189
Croll TP (2003) Bleaching sensitivity. JADA 134(9):1168
Cummins D (2009) Dentin hypersensitivity: from diagnosis to a breakthrough therapy for everyday sensitivity relief. J Clin Dent 20(Special Issue):1–9
Cummins D (2010) Recent advances in dentine hypersensitivity: clinical proven treatments for instant and lasting sensitivity relief. Am J Dent 23(Special Issue A 5):3A–13A
Cummins D (2011) Clinical evidence for the superior efficacy of a dentifrice containing 8.0% arginine and calcium carbonate in providing instant and lasting relief of dentin hypersensitivity. J Clin Dent 22(4):97–99
Cunha-Cruz J, Wataha JC, Zhou L, Manning W et al (2010) Treating dentin hypersensitivity therapeutic choices made by dentists of the Northwest PRECEDENT network. J Am Dent Assoc 141(9):1097–1105
Cunha-Cruz J, Stout JR, Heaton LJ, Wataha JC (2011) Dentin hypersensitivity and oxalates a systematic review. J Dent Res 90(3):304–310
Curro FA, Friedman M, Leight RS (2000) Design and conduct of clinical trials on dentine hypersensitivity. In: Addy M, Embery G, Edgar WM, Orchardson R (eds) Tooth wear and sensitivity. Clinical advances in restorative dentistry. Martin Dunitz Ltd, London, pp 299–314
Day TT, Einwag JJ, Hermann JS, He TT, Kay M et al (2010) A clinical assessment of the efficacy of a stannous-containing sodium fluoride dentifrice on dentinal hypersensitivity. J Contemp Dent Pract 11(1):E001–E008
de Assis CA, Antoniazzi RP, Zanatta FB, Rösing CK (2006) Efficacy of Gluma Desensitizer® on dentin hypersensitivity in periodontally treated patients. Braz Oral Res 20(3):252–256
Definition of active placebo (2013) www.thefreedictionary.com. Accessed 23 Apr 2013
Definition of nocebo effect (2013) http://www.medterms.com. Accessed 23 Apr 2013
Definition of placebo (2013) http://www.medterms.com. Accessed 23 Apr 2013
Docimo R, Montesani L, Maturo P, Costacurta M, Bartolino M, DeVizio W, Zhang YP, Cummins D, Dibart S, Mateo LR (2009) Comparing the efficacy in reducing dentin hypersensitivity of a new toothpaste containing 8.0%arginine, calcium carbonate, and 1450 ppm fluoride to a commercial sensitive toothpaste containing 2% potassium ion: An eight-week clinical study in Rome, Italy. J Clin Dent 20(Spec Iss):17–22
Dominiak M, Mierzwa D, Puzio M, Gedrange T (2012) Clinical evaluation of the effectiveness of using a collagen matrix (Mucograft® prototype) in gingival recession coverage-pilot study. J Stoma 65(2):184–197
Dondi dall'Orologio G, Malferrari S (1993) Desensitizing effects of Gluma and Gluma 2000 on hypersensitive dentin. Am J Dent 6(6):283–286
Dondi dall'Orologio G, Lorenzi R, Anselmi M, Opisso V (1999) Dentin desensitizing effects of Gluma Alternate, Health-Dent Desensitizer, and Scotchbond Multi-Purpose. Am J Dent 12(3):103–106
Dondi dall'Orologio G, Lone A, Finger WJ (2002) Clinical evaluation of the role of glutardialdehyde in a one-bottle adhesive. Am J Dent 15(5):330–334
Douglas de Oliveira DW, Oliveira-Ferreira F, Flecha OD, Gonçalves PF (2013) Is surgical root coverage effective for the treatment of cervical dentin hypersensitivity? A systematic review. J Periodontol 84(3):295–306
Drisko C (2002) Dentine hypersensitivity: dental hygiene and periodontal considerations. Int Dent J 52:385–393
Dunne SM, Hannington-Kiff JG (1993) The use of topical guanethidine in the relief of dentine hypersensitivity: a controlled study. Pain 54(2):165–168

Duran I, Sengun A (2004) The long-term effectiveness of five current desensitizing products on cervical dentine sensitivity. J Oral Rehabil 31:351–356
Ebisu S (2002) Calcium phosphate precipitation method for the treatment of dentin hypersensitivity. Am J Dent 15:220–226
Einwag J, Hermann J, He T, Day T, Zhang Y, Anastasia MK, Barker ML (2010) A clinical assessment of the efficacy of a stannous-containing sodium fluoride dentifrice on dentinal hypersensitivity. J Contemp Dent Pract 11:E001–E008, 26
Eitner S, Bittner C, Wichmann M, Nickenig HJ, Sokol B (2010) Comparison of conventional therapies for dentin hypersensitivity versus medical hypnosis. Int J Clin Exp Hypn 58(4):457–475
Felton DA, Bergenholtz G, Kanoy BE (1991) Evaluation of the desensitizing effect of Gluma Dentin Bond on teeth prepared for complete-coverage restorations. Int J Prosthodont 4(3):292–298
Ferrari M, Cagidiaco MC, Kugel G, Davidson CL (1999) Clinical evaluation of a one-bottle bonding system for desensitizing exposed roots. Am J Dent 12(5): 243–249
Francisconi LF, Scaffa PM, de Barros VR, Coutinho M, Francisconi PA (2009) Glass ionomer cements and their role in the restoration of non-carious cervical lesions. J Appl Oral Sci 17(5):364–369
Frechoso SC, Menéndez M, Guisasola C, Arregui I, Tejerina JM, Sicilia A (2003) Evaluation of the efficacy of two potassium nitrate bioadhesive gels (5% and 10%) in the treatment of dentine hypersensitivity. A randomised clinical trial. J Clin Periodontol 30(4):315–320
Froum S, Weinberg M, Novak J, Mailhot J et al (2004) A multicentre study evaluating the sensitization potential of enamel matrix derivative after treatment of two infrabony defects. J Periodontol 75:1001–1008
Furseth R (1970) A study of experimentally exposed and fluoride treated dental cementum in pigs. Acta Odontol Scand 28(6):833–850
Gaffar A (1999) Treating hypersensitivity with fluoride varnish. Compend Contin Educ Dent 20(1 Suppl): 27–33
Gandolfi MG, Taddei TA, Prati C (2010) Apatite-forming ability (bioactivity) of ProRoot MTA. Int Endod J 43(10):917–929
Gangarosa LP, Park NH (1978) Practical considerations in iontophoresis of fluoride for desensitizing dentin. J Prosthet Dent 39(2):173–178
Gedalia I, Brayer L, Katter N, Richter M, Stabholz A (1978) The effect of fluoride and strontium application on dentine. In vivo and in vitro studies. J Periodontol 49:269–272
Geiger S, Matalon S, Blasbalg J, Tung M, Eichmiller FC (2003) The clinical effect of amorphous calcium phosphate (ACP) on root surface hyper- sensitivity. Oper Dent 28:496–500
Gillam DG, Newman HN (1990) Iontophoresis in the treatment of cervical dentinal sensitivity–a review. J West Soc Periodontol Periodontal Abstr 38(4):129–133
Gillam DG (1992) The assessment and treatment of cervical dentinal sensitivity. DDS thesis, University of Edinburgh, Scotland
Gillam DG (1997) Clinical trial designs for testing of products for dentine hypersensitivity – a review. Periodontal Abstr 45:37–46
Gillam DG (2011) An overview on conducting clinical studies for the evaluation of desensitising products for the treatment of dentine hypersensitivity. Oral Health Dialog 2:6–14
Gillam DG, Orchardson R (2006) Advances in the treatment of root dentine sensitivity: mechanisms and treatment principles. Endod Topics 13:13–33
Gillam DG, Jackson RJ, Bulman JS, Newman HN (1996) Comparison of 2 desensitizing dentifrices with a commercially available fluoride dentifrice in alleviating cervical dentine sensitivity. J Periodontol 67:737–742
Gillam DG, Coventry J, Manning R, Newman HN, Bulman JS (1997a) Comparison of two desensitizing agents for the treatment of dentine hypersensitivity. Endod Dent Traumatol 13:36–39
Gillam DG, Mordan NJ, Newman HN (1997b) The Dentin Disc surface: a plausible model for dentin physiology and dentin sensitivity. Adv Dent Res 11(4):487–501
Gillam DG, Mordan NJ, Sinodinou AD, Tang JY et al (2001) The effects of oxalate-containing products on the exposed dentine surface: an SEM investigation. J Oral Rehabil 28:1037–1044
Gillam DG, Tang JY, Mordan NJ, Newman HN (2002) The effects of a novel Bioglass® dentifrice on dentine sensitivity: a scanning electron microscopy investigation. J Oral Rehabil 29(4):305–313
Gillam DG, Newman HN, Davies EH, Bulman JS, Troullos ES, Curro FA (2004) Clinical evaluation of ferric oxalate in relieving dentine hypersensitivity. J Oral Rehabil 31:245–250
Giniger M, Macdonald J, Ziemba S et al (2005) The clinical performance of professionally dispensed bleaching gel with added amorphous calcium phosphate. J Am Dent Assoc 136(3):383–392
Green BL, Green ML, McFall WT (1977) Calcium hydroxide and potassium nitrate as desensitizing agents for hypersensitive root surfaces. J Periodontol 48:667–672
Greene PR (1998) The flexible gingival mask: an aesthetic solution in periodontal practice. Br Dent J 184: 536–540
Greenhill JD, Pashley DH (1981) The effects of desensitizing agents on the hydraulic conductance of human dentin in vitro. J Dent Res 60(3):686–698
Gupta M, Pandit IK, Srivastava N, Gugnani N (2010) Comparative evaluation of 2% sodium fluoride iontophoresis and other cavity liners beneath silver amalgam restorations. J Indian Soc Pedod Prev Dent 28(2): 68–72
Gutentag H (1965) The effect of strontium chloride on peripheral nerve in comparison to the action of "stabilizer" and "labilizer" compounds. Penn Dent J (Phila) 68(2):37–43

Hamlin D, Williams KP, Delgado E, Zhang YP, DeVizio W, Mateo LR (2009) Clinical evaluation of the efficacy of a desensitizing paste containing 8% arginine and calcium carbonate for the in-office relief of dentin hypersensitivity associated with dental prophylaxis. Am J Dent 22(Sp Is A):16A–20A

Hannington-Kiff JG, Dunne SM (1993) Topical guanethidine relieves dentinal hypersensitivity and pain. J R Soc Med 86(9):514–515

Hansen EK (1992) Dentin hypersensitivity treated with a fluoride-containing varnish or a light-cured glass-ionomer liner. Eur J Oral Sci 100(6):305–309

Haywood VB (2000) Current status of night guard vital bleaching. Compend Contin Educ Dent 21(Suppl 28):S10–S17

Haywood VB (2002) Dentine hypersensitivity: bleaching and restorative considerations for successful management. Int Dent J 52(5):366–396

Haywood VB, Caughman F, Frazier KB, Myers ML (2001) Tray delivery of potassium nitrate-fluoride to reduce bleaching sensitivity. Quintessence Int 32:105–109

Haywood VB, Cordero R, Wright K, Gendreau L, Rupp R, Kotler M, Littlejohn S, Fabyanski J, Smith S (2005) Brushing with a potassium nitrate dentifrice to reduce bleaching sensitivity. J Clin Dent 16:17–22

Hazen SP, Volpe AR, King WJ (1968) Comparative desensitising effect of dentrifices containing sodium monofluorophosphate, stannous fluoride and formalin. Periodontics 6:230–232

He S, Wang Y, Li X, Hu D (2011) Effectiveness of laser therapy and topical desensitising agents in treating dentine hypersensitivity: a systematic review. J Oral Rehabil 38(5):348–358

Heard RH, Mellonig JT, Brunsvold MA, Lasho DJ et al (2000) Clinical evaluation of wound healing following multiple exposures to enamel matrix protein derivative in the treatment of infrabony periodontal defects. J Periodontol 71:1715–1721

Hench LL (2006) The story of Bioglass®. J Mater Sci Mater Med 17:967–978

Hill R, Gillam D, Karpukhina N (2012) The tubular occluding properties of a novel biomimetic hydroxyapatite toothpaste. In: Poster presentation (Abstr no. 640) IADR/PER Pan-European region meeting Helsinki, 12–15 Sept

Hoang-Dao BT, Hoang-Tu H, Tran-Thi N, Koubi G et al (2009) Clinical efficiency of a natural resin fluoride varnish (Shellac F) in reducing dentin hypersensitivity. J Oral Rehabil 36(2):124–131

Hodash M (1974) A superior desensitiser-potassium nitrate. J Am Dent Assoc 88:831–832

Holland GR, Narhi MN, Addy M, Gangarosa L, Orchardson R (1997) Guidelines for the design and conduct of clinical trials on dentine hypersensitivity. J Clin Periodontol 24:808–813

Homeopathic remedy for sensitive teeth (plantago). www.hpathy.com. Accessed 23 Apr 2013

Hróbjartsson A, Gøtzsche PC (2001) Is the placebo p? — An analysis of clinical trials comparing placebo with no treatment. N Engl J Med 344:1594–1602

http://www.medterms.com. Accessed 23 Apr 2013

Hughes N, Mason S, Jeffery P et al (2010) A comparative clinical study investigating the efficacy of a test dentifrice containing 8% strontium acetate and 1040 ppm sodium fluoride versus a marketed control dentifrice containing 8% arginine, calcium carbonate, and 1450 ppm sodium monofluorophosphate in reducing dentinal hypersensitivity. J Clin Dent 21(2):49–55

Ilnyckyj A, Shanahan F, Anton PA, Cheang M, Bernstein CN (1997) Quantification of the placebo response in ulcerative colitis. Gastroenterology 112:1854–1858

Ipci SD, Cakar G, Kuru B, Yilmaz S (2009) Clinical evaluation of lasers and sodium fluoride gel in the treatment of dentine hypersensitivity. Photomed Laser Surg 27(1):85–91

Jackson RJ (2000) Potential treatment modalities for dentine hypersensitivity: home use products. In: Addy M, Embery G, Edgar WM, Orchardson R (eds) Tooth wear and sensitivity. Clinical advances in restorative dentistry. Martin Dunitz, London, pp 327–338

Jeffcott M (1993) Chemical plaque control: how do you advise your patients? Int Dent J 43:415–421

Kakaboura A, Rahiotis C, Thomaidis S, Doukoudakis S (2005) Clinical effectiveness of two agents on the treatment of tooth cervical hypersensitivity. Am Dent J 18(4):291–295

Kang S-J KY-H, Park J-B Herr Y, Chung J-H (2009) The effects of hydroxyapatite toothpaste on tooth hypersensitivity. J Korean Acad Periodontol 39:9–16 (Korean)

Kara C, Orbak R (2009) Comparative evaluation of Nd:YAG laser and fluoride varnish for the treatment of dentinal hypersensitivity. J Endod 35(7):971–974

Karim BFA, Gillam DG (2013) The efficacy of strontium and potassium toothpastes in treating dentine hypersensitivity: a systematic review. Int J Dent 2013(2013), Article ID 573258, 13 p. http://dx.doi.org/10.1155/2013/573258

Kawasaki A, Ishikawa K, Suge T, Shimizu H et al (2001) Effects of plaque control on the patency and occlusion of dentine tubules in situ. J Oral Rehabil 28:439–449

Kerns DG, Scheidt MJ, Pashley DH, Horner JA, Strong SL, Van Dyke TE (1991) Dentinal tubule occlusion and root hypersensitivity. J Periodontol 62:421–428

Kielbassa AM, Attin T, Hellwig E, Schade-Brittinger C (1997) In vivo study on the effectiveness of a lacquer containing CaF2/NaF in treating dentine hypersensitivity. Clin Oral Invest 1:95–99

Kim S (1986) Hypersensitive teeth. Desensitization of pulpal sensory nerves. J Endod 12:482–485

Kim SH, Park JB, Lee CW, Koo KT, Kim TI, Seol YJ et al (2009) The clinical effects of a hydroxyapatite containing toothpaste for dentine hypersensitivity. J Korean Acad Periodontol 39(1):87–94 (Korean)

Kimura Y, Wilder-Smith P, Yonaga K, Matsumoto K (2000) Treatment of dentine hypersensitivity by lasers: a review. J Clin Periodontol 27:715–721

Kleinberg I (2002) SensiStat, a new saliva-based composition for simple and effective treatment of entinal sensitivity pain. Dent Today 21:42–47

Kolker JL, Vargas MA, Armstrong SR, Dawson DV (2002) Effect of desensitizing agents on dentin permeability and dentin tubule occlusion. J Adhes Dent 4(3):211–221

Kun L (1976) Biophsical study of dental tissues under the effect of a local strontium application Schweiz Monatsschr Zahnheilkd. 86(7):661–76. [Article in French]

Leonard RH, Smith LR, Garland GE, Caplan DJ (2004) Desensitising agent efficacy during whitening in an at-risk population. J Esthet Restor Dent 16(1):49–55; discussion 56

Li Y, Lee S, Mateo LR, Delgado E, Zhang YP (2013) Comparison of clinical efficacy of three professionally applied pastes on immediate and sustained reduction of dentin hypersensitivity. Compend Contin Educ Dent 34(1):6–12 (online access 10 May 2013)

Lin YH, Gillam DG (2012) The prevalence of root sensitivity following periodontal therapy: a systematic review. Int J Dent 2012:407023. doi:10.1155/2012/407023, Epub 2012 Oct 31

Lin PY, Cheng YW, Chu CY, Chien KL, Lin CP, Tu YK (2013) In-office treatment for dentin hypersensitivity: a systematic review and network meta-analysis. J Clin Periodontol 40:53–64

Ling TYY, Gillam DG (1996) The effectiveness of desensitizing agents for the treatment of cervical dentine sensitivity (CDS) – a review. Periodontal Abstr 44(1):5–12

Litkowski LJ, Quinlan KB, McDonald NJ (1998) Teeth hypersensitivity reduction by a novel Bioglass® dentifrice. J Dent Res 77(Suppl 1):199

Love RM, Jenkinson HF (2002) Invasion of dentinal Tubules by oral bacteria. Crit Rev Oral Biol Med 13(2):171–183

Low T (1981) The treatment of hypersensitive cervical abrasion cavities using ASPA cement. J Oral Rehabil 8(1):81–89

Lukomsky EH (1941) Fluoride therapy for exposed dentin and alveolar atrophy. J Dent Res 20:649–654

Mahmound AS, Almas K, Dahlan Al-Raheem AA (1999) The effect of propolis on dentinal hypersensitivity and level of satisfaction among patients from a university hospital Riyadh, Saudi Arabia. Indian J Dent Res 10:130–137

Markowitz K (2010) Pretty painful: why does tooth bleaching hurt? Med Hypotheses 74(5):835–840

Markowitz K, Kim S (1985) The effects of various ionic solutions on pulpal nerve sensitivity. J Dent Res 64:309 (Abstr no. 1213)

Markowitz K, Kim S (1990) Hypersensitive teeth. Experimental studies of dentinal desensitizing agents. Dent Clin North Am 34(3):491–501. Review

Markowitz K, Nârhi M, Ngassapa D, Kim S (1990) The effect of KCl on intradental nerve activity evoked by hypertonic NaCl solution and natural stimuli ¡abstract 1492. J Dent Res 69(special issue 1):295

Markowitz K, Bilotto G, Kim S (1991) Decreasing intradental nerve activity in the cat with potassium and divalent cations. Arch Oral Biol 36:1–7

Mason S, Hughes N, Sufi F, Bannon L, Maggio B, North M, Holt J (2010) A comparative clinical study investigating the efficacy of a dentifrice containing 8% strontium acetate and 1040 ppm fluoride in a silica base and a control dentifrice containing 1450 ppm fluoride in a silica base to provide immediate relief of dentin hypersensitivity. J Clin Dent 21(Spec Iss):42–48

McCarthy D, Gillam DG, Parson DJ (1997) In vitro effects of laser radiation on dentine surfaces. J Dent Res 76(Special issue):233

McCormack K, Davies R (1996) The enigma of potassium ion in the management of dentine hypersensitivity: is nitric oxide the elusive second messenger? Pain 68:5–11

McFall WT (1986) A review of active agents available for the treatment of dentinal hypersensitivity. Endod Dent Traumatol 2:141–149

Mehmood Z, Shah JA, Javed MU, Manzoor MA et al (2011) Efficacy of GLUMA desensitizer® and Duraphat™ in relieving dentinal hypersensitivity in non-carious cervical lesions. Pak Oral Dent J 31(1): 183–186

Merika K, Hefti AF, Preshaw PM (2006) Comparison of two topical treatments for dentin sensitivity. Eur Prosthodont Restor Dent 14(1):38–41

Milleman JL et al (2012) NUPRO Sensodyne prophylaxis paste with NovaMin for the treatment of dentin hypersensitivity: a 4-week clinical study. Am J Dent 25:262–268

Miller PD Jr (1985) A classification of marginal tissue recession. Int J Periodontics Restorative Dent 5:9–13

Miller JT, Shannon IL, Kilgore WG, Bookman JE (1969) Use of a water-free stannous fluoride-containing gel in the control of dental hypersensitivity. J Periodontol 40(8):490–491

Mneimne M, Hill RG, Bushby AJ, Brauer DS (2011) High phosphate content significantly increases apatite formation of fluoride-containing bioactive glasses. Acta Biomater 7:1827–1834

Mordan NJ, Gillam DG, Critchell J, Curro FA, Ley F (2002) Effects of abrasive components on dentine: an SEM study. IADR meeting San Diego, Poster abstract no. 3010

Morris MF, Davis RD, Richardson BW (1999) Clinical efficacy of two dentin desensitizing agents. Am J Dent 12:72–76

Mostafa P, Addy M, Morgan T (1983) Scanning electron-microscopic, X-ray diffraction analysis, atomic absorption and fluoride probe measurements of the uptake of toothpaste ingredients onto dentine. J Dent Res 62:433 (Abstr no. 165)

Mount GJ, Tyas MJ, Ferracane JL, Nicholson JW et al (2009) A revised classification for direct tooth-colored restorative materials. Quintessence Int 40(8):691–697

Muzzin KB, Johnson R (1989) Effects of potassium oxalate on dentin hypersensitivity in vivo. J Periodontol 60:151–158

Nathoo S, Delgado E, Zhang YP, DeVizio W, Cummins D, Mateo LR (2009) Comparing the efficacy in providing instant relief of dentin hypersensitivity of a new toothpaste containing 8.0% arginine, calcium carbonate, and 1450 ppm fluoride to a benchmark, desensitizing toothpaste containing 2% potassium ion and 1450ppm fluoride, and to a control toothpaste with 1450ppm fluoride. A three–day clinical study in New Jersey, USA. J Clin Dent 20:123–130

Neuhaus KW, Milleman JL, Milleman KR, Mongiello KA et al (2013) Effectiveness of a calcium sodium phosphosilicate containing prophylaxis paste in reducing dentine hypersensitivity immediately and 4 weeks after a single application: a double-blind randomized controlled trial. J Clin Periodontol 40(4): 349–357

Ni LX, He T, Chang A, Sun L (2010) The desensitizing efficacy of a novel stannous-containing sodium fluoride dentifrice: an 8-week randomized and controlled clinical trial. Am J Dent 23(Sp Is B):17B–21B

Nishida M, Katamsi D, Uchida A et al (1976) Hypersensitivity of the exposed root surfaces after surgical periodontal treatment. J Osaka Univ Dent Soc 16:73–77

Oken BS (2008) Placebo effects: clinical aspects and neurobiology. Brain 131:2812–2823

Ong G, Strahan JD (1989) Effect of a desensitizing dentifrice on dentinal hypersensitivity. Endod Dent Traumatol 5:213–218

Orchardson R, Gillam D (2000) The efficacy of potassium salts as agents for treating dentin hypersensitivity. J Orofac Pain 14(1):9–19

Orchardson R, Gillam D (2006) Managing dentin hypersensitivity. J Am Dent Assoc 137(7):990–998

Orchardson R, Peacock JM, Whitters CJ (1997) Effect of pulsed Nd:YAG laser radiation on action potential conduction in isolated mammalian spinal nerves. Lasers Surg Med 21(2):142–148

Orchardson R, Peacock JM, Whitters CJ (1998) Effects of pulsed Nd:YAG laser radiation on action potential conduction in nerve fibres inside teeth in vitro. J Dent 26:421–426

Orsini G, Procaccini M, Manzoli L, Giuliodori F, Lorenzini A, Putignano A (2010) A double-blind randomized-controlled trial comparing the desensitizing efficacy of a new dentifrice containing carbonate/hydroxyl- apatite nanocrystals and a sodium fluoride/potassium nitrate dentifrice. J Clin Periodontol 37:510–517

Özgünaltay G, Önen A (2002) Three-year clinical evaluation of a resin modified glass–ionomer cement and a composite resin in non-carious class V lesions. J Oral Rehabil 29:1037–1041

Pagliaro U, Nieri M, Franceschi D, Clauser C, Pini-Prato G (2003) Evidenced-based mucogingival therapy. Part 1: a critical review of the literature on root coverage procedures. J Periodontol 74:709–740

Paine ML, Slots J, Rich SK (1998) Fluoride use in periodontal therapy: a review of the literature. J Am Dent Assoc 129:69–76

Pamir T, Dalgar H, Onal B (2007) Clinical evaluation of three desensitizing agents in relieving dentin hypersensitivity. Oper Dent 32:544–548

Pandurić V, Knežević A, Tarle Z, Šutalo J (2001) The efficiency of dentine adhesives in treating non-caries cervical lesions. J Oral Rehabil 28(12):1168–1174

Pardi V, Pereira AC, Mialhe FL, Meneghim Mde C, Ambrosano GM (2003) A 5-year evaluation of two glass-ionomer cements used as fissure sealants. Community Dent Oral Epidemiol 31(5):386–391

Park JJ, Park JB, Kwon YH, Herr Y, Chung JH (2005) The effect of microcrystalline hydroxyapatite containing toothpaste in the control of tooth hypersensitivity. J Korean Acad Periodontol 35:577–590

Pashely DH, Tay FR, Haywood HB et al (2008) Consensus-based recommendations for the diagnosis and management of dentin hypersensitivity. Comp Contin Educ Dent 29(8 Suppl):1S–35S

Pashley DH (1992a) Dentin permeability and dentin sensitivity. Proc Finn Dent Soc 88(Suppl 1):215–224

Pashley DH (1992b) Dentin bonding agents. Curr Opin Dent 2:46–51

Pashley DH (2000) Potential treatment modalities for dentine hyper- sensitivity: in-office products. In: Addy M, Embery G, Edgar WM, Orchardson R (eds) Tooth wear and sensitivity. Martin Dunitz, London, pp 351–365

Pashley DH (1984) Smear layer: physiological considerations. Oper Dent Suppl 3:13–29

Pashley DH, Kalathoor S, Burnham D (1986) The effects of calcium hydroxide on dentin permeability. J Dent Res 65(3):417–420

Pashley DH, Carvalho RM, Pereira JC, Villanueva R, Tay FR (2001) The use of oxalate to reduce dentin permeability under adhesive restorations. Am J Dent 14:89–94

Paternak MA, Zimmerman M (2007) Therapeutic effect of follow-up assessments on antidepressant and placebo response rates in antidepressant efficacy trials. Br J Psychiatry 190:287–292

Pawlowska J (1956) Strontium chloride its importance in dentistry and prophylaxis. Czas Stomal 9:353–361

Pearce N, Addy M, Newcombe RG (1994) Dentine hypersensitivity: a clinical trial to compare 2 strontium desensitising toothpastes with a conventional fluoride toothpaste. J Periodontol 65:113–119

Petrou I, Heu R, Stranick M, Lavender S, Zaidel L, Cummins D, Sullivan RJ, Hsueh C, Gimzewski JK (2009) A breakthrough therapy for dentin hypersensitivity: how dental products containing 8% arginine and calcium carbonate work to deliver effective relief of sensitive teeth. J Clin Dent 20(Spec Iss):23–31

Pillon FL, Romani IG, Schmidt ER (2004) Effect of a 3% potassium oxalate topical application on dentinal hypersensitivity after subgingival scaling and root planing. J Periodontol 75:1461–1464

Pol DG, Jonnala J, Chute M, Gunjikar T, Pol S (2010) Potassium nitrate in the treatment of dentinal hypersensitivity- a mini analysis of studies. JIDA 4:399–403

Polderman RN, Frencken JE (2007) Comparison between effectiveness of a low-viscosity glass ionomer and a resin-based glutaraldehyde containing primer in

treating dentine hypersensitivity-a 25.2-month evaluation. J Dent 35:144–149
Porto ICCM (2012) Post-operative sensitivity in direct resin composite restorations: clinical practice guidelines. IJRD 1:1–12
Poulsen S, Errboe M, Lescay Mevil Y, and Glenny A-M (2006) Potassium containing toothpastes for dentine hypersensitivity. Cochrane Database Syst Rev (Issue 3). Art no. CD001476. doi:10.1002/14651858.CD001476.pub2
Pradeep AR, Sharma A (2010) Comparison of clinical efficacy of a dentifrice containing calcium sodium phosphosilicate to a dentifrice containing potassium nitrate and to a placebo on dentinal hypersensitivity: a randomized clinical trial. J Periodontol 81(8):1167–1173
Prati C, Cervellati F, Sanasi V, Montebugnoli L (2001) Treatment of cervical dentin hypersensitivity with resin adhesives: 4-week evaluation. Am J Dent 14(6):378–382
Que K, Fu Y, Lin L, Hu D, Zhang YP, Panagakos FS et al (2010) Dentin hypersensitivity reduction of new toothpaste containing 8.0% arginine and 1450 ppm fluoride: an 8-week clinical study on Chinese adults. Am J Dent 23A(Special Issue):28A–35A
Renton-Harper P, Midda M (1992) NdYAG laser treatment of dentinal hypersensitivity. Br Dent J 172(1): 13–16
Reynolds EC (1998) Anticariogenic complexes of amorphous calcium phosphate stabilized by casein phosphopeptides: a review. Spec Care Dentist 18(1):8–16
Rimondini L, Palazzo B, Iafisco M, Canegallo F et al (2007) The remineralizing effect of a carbonate-hydroxyapatite microparticles on dentine on dentine. Mater Sci Forum 539:602–605
Ritter AV, de Dias WL, Miguez P, Caplan DJ et al (2006) Treating cervical dentin hypersensitivity with fluoride varnish a randomized clinical study. JADA 137:1013–1020
Ross MR (1961) Hypersensitive teeth: effect of strontium chloride in a compatible dentifrice. J Periodontol 32:49–53
Saadoun AP (2008) Root coverage with Emdogain/Alloderm: a new way to treat gingival recessions. Eur J Esthet Dent 3(1):46–65
Salvato A, Troullos ES, Curro FA, Merola MR et al (1990) The effectiveness of Ferric Oxalate (FO) in relieving dentinal hypersensitivity. J Dent Res 69 (Special Issue):169 (Abstr no. 482)
Sandoval E, Shannon IL (1969) Stannous fluoride and dentin solubility. Tex Rep Biol Med 27(1):111–116
Santamaria MP, Suaid FF, Nociti FH Jr, Zaffalon M et al (2007) Periodontal surgery and glass ionomer restoration in the treatment of gingival recession associated with a non-carious cervical lesion: report of three cases. J Periodontol 78(6):1146–1153
Sanz M, Lorenzo R, Aranda JJ, Martin C et al (2009) Clinical evaluation of a new collagen matrix (Mucograft ® prototype) to enhance the width of keratinized tissue in patients with fixed prosthetic restorations: a randomized prospective clinical trial. J Periodontol 36:868–876
Schiff T, Saletta L, Baker RA, Winston JL, He T (2005) Desensitizing effect of a stabilized stannous fluoride/sodium hexametaphosphate dentifrice. Compend Contin Educ Dent 26(Supp 1):35–40
Schiff T, He T, Sagel L, Baker R (2006) Efficacy and safety of a novel stabilized stannous fluoride and sodium hexametaphosphate dentifrice for dentinal hypersensitivity. J Contemp Dent Pract 7(2):1–008
Schiff T, Delgado E, Zhang YP, DeVizio W, Mateo LR (2009a) Clinical evaluation of the efficacy of a desensitizing paste containing 8% arginine and calcium carbonate in providing instant and lasting in-office relief of dentin hypersensitivity. Am J Dent 22(Sp Is A):8A–15A
Schiff T, Delgado E, Zhang YP, DeVizio W, Cummins D, Mateo LR (2009b) The clinical effect of a single direct topical application of a dentifrice containing 8.0% arginine, calcium carbonate, and 1450 ppm fluoride on dentin hypersensitivity: the use of a cotton swab applicator versus the use of a fingertip. J Clin Dent 20(4):131–136
Schiff T, Mateo LR, Delgado E, Cummins D, Zhang YP, DeVizio W (2011) Clinical efficacy in reducing dentin hypersensitivity of a dentifrice containing 8.0% arginine, calcium carbonate, and 1450 ppm fluoride compared to a dentifrice containing 8% strontium acetate and 1040 ppm fluoride under consumer usage conditions before and after switch-over. J Clin Dent 22(4):128–138
Schwarz F, Arweller N, Georg T, Reich E (2002) Desensitizing effects of an Er:YAG laser on hypersensitive dentine: a controlled, prospective clinical study. J Clin Periodontol 29(3):211–215
Sena FJ (1990) Dentinal permeability in assessing therapeutic agents. Dent Clin North Am 34(3):475–490
Sgolastra F, Petrucci A, Severino M, Gatto R, Monaco A (2013) Lasers for the treatment of dentin hypersensitivity: a meta-analysis J Dent Res 92(6)492–9. doi: 10.1177/0022034513487212.[Epub 2013 Apr 22].
Sharif MO, Iram S, Brunton PA (2013) Effectiveness of arginine-containing toothpastes in treating dentine hypersensitivity: a systematic review. J Dent 41(6):483–492
Sharma AA, Park JH (2010) Esthetic considerations in interdental papilla: remediation and regeneration. J Esthet Restor Dent 22:18–30, _307 18
Sicilia A, Cuesta-Frechoso S, Suarez A, Angulo J et al (2009) Immediate efficacy of diode laser application in the treatment of dentine hypersensitivity in periodontal maintenance patients: a randomized clinical trial. J Clin Periodontol 36(8):650–660
Skurnik H (1963) Control of dental hypersensitivity: preliminary report on a strontium containing dentifrice. J Periodontol 34:183
Starr CB, Mayhew RB, Pierson WP (1989) The efficacy of hypnosis in the treatment of dentin hypersensitivity. Gen Dent 37:13–15
Stead WJ, Orchardson R, Warren PB (1996) A mechanical model of potassium ion diffusion in dentinal tubules. Arch Oral Biol 41:679–687
Stewardson DA, Crisp RJ, McHugh S, Lendenmann U, Burke FJ (2004) The Effectiveness of Systemp.

desensitizer in the treatment of dentine hypersensitivity. Prim Dent Care 11(3):71–76
Suge T, Ishikawa K, Kawasaki A, Suzuki K, Matsuo T, Noiri Y, Imazato S (2002) Calcium phosphate precipitation method for the treatment of dentin hypersensitivity. Am J Dent 15:220–226
Swift EJ Jr, May KN Jr, Mitchell S (2001) Clinical evaluation of Prime & Bond 2.1 for treating cervical dentin hypersensitivity. Am J Dent 14(1):13–16
Swift EJ (2005) Tooth sensitivity and whitening. Compend Contin Educ Dent 26(9 Suppl 3):4–10; quiz 23
Tai BJ, Bian Z, Jiang H, Greenspan DC, Zhong J, Clark AE, Du MQ (2006) Anti-gingivitis effect of a dentifrice containing bioactive glass (NovaMin®) particulate. J Clin Periodontol 33(2):86–91
Tammaro S, Wennstrom JL, Bergenholtz G (2000) Root-dentin sensitivity following non-surgical periodontal treatment. J Clin Periodontol 27:690–697
Tantbirojn D, Poolthong S, Leevailoj C, Srisawasdi S et al (2006) Clinical evaluation of a resin-modified glass-ionomer liner for cervical dentin hypersensitivity treatment. Am J Dent 19(1):56–60
Tay FR, Pashley DH, Mak YF, Carvalho RM, Lai SC, Suh BI (2003) Integrating oxalate desensitizers with total-etch two-step adhesive. J Dent Res 82:703–707
Thrash WJ, Jones DL, Dodds WJ (1992) Effect of a fluoride solution on dentinal hypersensitivity. Am J Dent 5:299–302
Tjan AHL, Chan CAC (1987) Effects of resin-compatible cavity varnishes on the polymerization of visible light cured composites. J Prosthet Dent 58:559–563
Tjan AHL, Grant BE, Nemetz H (1987) The efficacy of resin-compatible cavity varnishes in reducing dentin permeability to free monomer. J Prosthet Dent 57:179–185
Tredwin CJ, Naik S, Lewis NJ, Scully C (2006) Hydrogen peroxide tooth-whitening (bleaching) products: review of adverse effects and safety issues. Br Dent J 200(7):371–376
Tschoppe P, Zandim DL, Martus P, Kielbassa AM (2011) Enamel and dentine remineralization by nano-hydroxyapatite toothpastes. J Dent 39:430–437
Tugnait A, Clerehugh V (2001) Gingival recession-its significance and management. J Dent 29:381–394
Tyas MJ, Burrow MF (2004) Adhesive restorative materials: a review. Aust Dent J 49(3):112–121
Uchida A, Wakano Y, Fukuyama O, Miki T, Iwayama Y, Okada H (1980) Controlled clinical evaluation of a 10% strontium chloride dentifrice in treatment of dentin hypersensitivity following periodontal surgery. J Periodontol 51:578–581
Umberto R, Claudia R, Gaspare P, Tenore G, Alessandro DV (2012) Treatment of dentine hypersensitivity by diode laser: a clinical study. Int J Dent Article ID 858950, 8 pages
Veitz-Keenan A, Barna JA, Strober B, Matthews AG et al (2013) Treatments for hypersensitive noncarious cervical lesions: a Practitioners Engaged in Applied Research and Learning (PEARL) Network randomized clinical effectiveness study. J Am Dent Assoc 144(5):495–506
Vollenweider M, Brunner TJ, Knecht S, Grass RN, Zehnder M, Imfeld T, Stark WJ (2007) Remineralization of human dentin using ultrafine bioactive glass particles. Acta Biomater 3:936–943
von Troil BV, Needleman I, Sanz M (2002) A systematic review of the prevalence of root sensitivity following periodontal therapy. J Clin Periodontol 29(Suppl 3):173–177
Voth ED, Phillips RW, Swartz ML (1966) Thermal diffusion through amalgam and various liners. J Dent Res 45:1184–1190
Wallace JA, Bissada NF (1990) Pulpal and root sensitivity rated to periodontal therapy. Oral Surg Oral Med Oral Pathol 69:743–747
Walsh LJ (2010) The effects of GC Tooth Mousse on cervical dentinal sensitivity: a controlled clinical trial. Int Dent SA 12(1):4–12
Wang H-L, Yeh C-T, Smith F, Burgett FG et al (1993) Evaluation of ferric oxalate as an agent for use during surgery to prevent post-operative root hypersensitivity. J Periodontol 64(11):1040–1044
Wang ZJ, Sa Y, Sauro S, Chen H, Xing WZ, Ma X et al (2010) Effect of desensitising toothpastes on dentinal tubule occlusion: a dentine permeability measurement and SEM in vitro study. J Dent 38(5):400–410
West NX (2007) The dentine hypersensitivity patient – a total management package. Int Dent J 57(Suppl 1):411–419
West NX, Addy M, Jackson RJ, Ridge DB (1997) Dentine hypersensitivity and the placebo response. A comparison of strontium acetate, potassium nitrate and fluoride toothpastes. J Clin Periodontol 24:209–215
Wolfart S, Wegner SM, Kern M (2004) Comparison of using calcium hydroxide or a dentine primer for reducing dentinal pain following crown preparation: a randomized clinical trial with an observation time up to 30 months. J Oral Rehabil 31(4):344–350
www.thefreedictionary.com. Accessed 23 Apr 2013
Wycoff SJ (1982) Current treatment for dentinal hypersensitivity. In-office treatment. Compend Contin Educ Dent (Suppl 3):S113–5
Yilmaz HG, Kurtulmus-Yilmaz S, Cengiz E, Bayindir H, Aykac Y (2011a) Clinical evaluation of Er, Cr:YSGG and GaAlAs laser therapy for treating dentine hypersensitivity: a randomized controlled clinical trial. J Dent 39(3):249–254
Yilmaz HG, Cengiz E, Kurtulmus-Yilmaz S, Leblebicioglu B (2011b) Effectiveness of Er, Cr:YSGG laser on dentine hypersensitivity: a controlled clinical trial. J Clin Periodontol 38(4):341–346
Yan B, Yi J, Li Y, Chen Y, Shi Z (2013) Arginine-containing toothpastes for dentin hypersensitivity: systematic review and meta-analysis. Quintessence Int 44(9):709–723
Yiu CKY, King NM, Suh BI, Sharp LJ et al (2005) Incompatibility of oxalate desensitizers with acidic, fluoride-containing total-etch adhesives. J Dent Res 84(8):730–735
Yuan P, Shen X, Liu J, Hou Y, Zhu M et al (2012) Effects of dentifrice containing hydroxyapatite on dentinal

tubule occlusion and hexavalent chromium cations sorption: a preliminary study. PLoS ONE 7(12):e45283. doi:10.1371/journal.pone.0045283
Zaher CA, Hachem J, Puhan MA, Mombelli A (2005) Interest in periodontology and preferences for treatment of localized gingival recessions. A survey among Swiss dentists. J Clin Periodontol 32:375–382
Zalkind M, Hochman N (1997) Alternative method of conservative aesthetic treatment for gingival recession. J Prosthet Dent 77:561–563
Zetterstrom O, Andersson C, Eriksson L, Fredriksson A et al (1997) Clinical safety of enamel matrix derivative (EMDOGAIN) in the treatment of periodontal defects. J Clin Periodontol 24(Part 2):697–704

Treatment Modalities for Dentin Hypersensitivity

6

David G. Gillam

Abstract

The aim of this chapter is to provide the dental professional with the necessary information in order to treat dentin hypersensitivity by using selected at-home and in-office products with an emphasis on developing a workable maintenance programme which will enable the dental professional to effectively manage this troublesome clinical condition.

6.1 Introduction

A number of in-office and at-home or over-the-counter (OTC) desensitising products have been employed by dental professionals in order to alleviate dentin hypersensitivity (DH), and these have been classified by a number of investigators based either on anti-inflammatory drugs, protein precipitants, tubular occluding agents and tubular sealants or on their physical or chemical properties (Ong 1986; Scherman and Jacobsen 1992). However, neither of these classifications may be considered to be ideal since they fail to take into account the products that act to block pulpal nerve activity by direct ionic diffusion or procedures such as hypnosis or hypnotherapy. More recent classifications, however, are based on whether they are in-office or over-the-counter (OTC) products or procedures (Gillam 1997; Pashley 2000). A further classification has also been considered by Haywood (2002) who proposed a simple classification of reversible and nonreversible agents, restorative materials and procedures. More recently, Gillam and Turner (2013) proposed a classification in relation to the treatment of gingival recession with associated DH, for example, based on nonsurgical and surgical approaches.

According to Grossman (1935) an ideal desensitising agent or technique should fulfill the following criteria:

1. It should not unduly irritate nor in any way endanger the integrity of the pulp.
2. It should be relatively painless on application or shortly afterwards.
3. It should be easily applied.
4. It should be rapid in its action.
5. It should be permanently effective.
6. It should not discolour tooth substance.

Gillam (1997) however suggested that these recommendations should be updated in the following manner:

D.G. Gillam
Centre for Adult Oral Health,
Institute of Dentistry, Barts and the London
School of Medicine and Dentistry QMUL,
Turner Street, London E1 2AD, UK
e-mail: d.g.gillam@qmul.ac.uk

S. Taha, B.H. Clarkson (eds.), *Clinician's Guide to the Diagnosis and Management of Tooth Sensitivity*,
DOI 10.1007/978-3-642-45164-5_6, © Springer-Verlag Berlin Heidelberg 2014

1. An OTC product should meet the following criteria:
   (a) Be effective in the desired mode of delivery. Product A might be effective as a paste but not in a mouthwash.
   (b) Be able to exert its effect over time to give relief from pain and/or prevent further attacks.
   (c) Be safe to use.
   (d) Be demonstrably effective in well-controlled clinical studies.
   (e) Have substantiated claims of efficacy regarding proposed usage.
   (f) Have the correct marketing appeal for the population targeted. Is it in a form (gel or paste) that is pleasant to taste and effective in its claims, e.g. relieves or prevents pain (quickly cleans teeth, etc.)?
   (g) Satisfy the subject with the outcome of treatment.
2. An in-office product should meet the following criteria:
   (a) Be effective in the desired mode of delivery
   (b) Be able to exert its effect immediately to give relief from pain and/or prevent further attacks
   (c) Be safe to use and not stain teeth or induce adverse pulpal changes
   (d) Be demonstrably effective in well-controlled clinical studies
   (e) Have substantiated claims of efficacy regarding proposed modes of action
   (f) Be easy to apply and painless
   (g) Satisfy the subject with the outcome of treatment

Neither recommendation, however, specifically addresses the problem of the quality of life dimension that can be problematic for the patient (Bekes et al. 2009; Gibson et al. 2010).

Currently there is a plethora of remedies available for both OTC and in-office applications; however, it is evident that none of these products appear to provide an effective long-lasting solution to the problem (Canadian Advisory Board on Dentin Hypersensitivity 2003; Orchardson and Gillam 2006). Most of these products work either on the basis of their tubular occluding properties, for example, strontium-based (chloride, acetate) products or by nerve desensitisation, for example, potassium-based (chloride, citrate, nitrate) products. Evidence for their efficacy however has been questioned by several investigators in a series of reviews over the last decade (Zappa 1994; Jackson 2000; Orchardson and Gillam 2000; Poulsen et al. 2006; Cummins 2009, 2010; Karim and Gillam 2013). It is also important to recognise the claims that have been made for these products, and these are generally based on whether the product has an immediate action in relieving DH or is long-lasting in its effect. Generally speaking it would be reasonable to expect an in-office product to have an immediate effect following application, whereas a toothpaste product may take 2–4 weeks of tooth brushing in order to achieve an effect. The problem however with these claims is that one cannot always substantiate the claim from the actual study. For example, if a claim of immediate relief is made, one would expect within 5–10 min following application and subsequent testing that there would be relief; however, one could not make this claim if the testing was performed after 24 h. When making a claim that a product has a long-lasting effect, then short-term studies up to 6 weeks may not be sufficient to make this claim. Ideally studies that claim a long-lasting effect would need to be of a longer duration in order to make such a claim.

Products designed to alleviate DH are generally produced in formulations that can be either applied 'in office' such as varnishes, gels, desensitising polishing pastes and dentin bonding agents or purchased over the counter (OTC) for at-home use (e.g. dentifrices, gels, mouthwashes and chewing gums). Other treatments such as laser therapy and hypnosis/hypnotherapy have also been reported in the literature (Starr et al. 1989; Eitner et al. 2010). It should however be mentioned that root canal therapy and extraction of the offending tooth or teeth may also be a treatment option depending on the prognosis of the tooth (Gillam 1992).

6.2 Prevention of Tooth Sensitivity

Prior to considering any treatment, however, it is essential for the dental professional to appreciate that DH is essentially a diagnosis of exclusion, and it is incumbent on the dental professional to consider initiating a differential diagnosis in order to determine the exact cause of the patient's pain. For example, the patient's discomfort may be due to pain from caries, fractured teeth or post-operative pain from restorative procedures (fillings, periodontal treatment, bleaching). In order for any subsequent treatment to be effective, identification of the exact cause of the pain is imperative, and this may involve time-consuming investigations including sensibility (sensitivity) testing and radiographic investigation. Identification of DH may be made by the dental professional using cold air from a dental air syringe and an explorer probe. A useful tip in diagnosing DH may be the application of a varnish, for example, Duraphat, on the exposed root surface with the clinician evaluating the severity of the problem before and after application with an air blast from a dental air syringe. It is however important to note that simply treating the problem without any consideration of the aetiological and predisposing factors associated with the initiation of DH will not necessarily prevent the problem reoccurring in the future. Successful management of the problem of DH therefore must include preventive strategies, irrespective of any treatment recommended or provided by the dental professional (Drisko 2002; Gillam and Orchardson 2006; Orchardson and Gillam 2006).

A management strategy should be based on the extent and severity of the problem (localised/generalised) and treated accordingly. For example, localised problems may be treated in office using primers, varnishes, sealants, glass ionomer cements, composite restorations whereas a mild/moderate generalised problem may be treated with over-the-counter products such as toothpaste formulation containing strontium or potassium salts (Orchardson and Gillam 2006). According to Gillam and Orchardson (2006), a number of aetiological and predisposing factors that may be involved in the exposure of the dentin have been identified, for example, attrition, abrasion, abfraction, erosion, gingival recession, quality of the buccal bone, periodontal disease and its treatment, surgical and restorative procedures and patient destructive habits. Dababneh et al. (1999) also reported that the aetiological factors associated with DH may bring about two specific biological processes in the affected tooth, namely, lesion localisation and lesion initiation. Lesion localisation occurs when the dentin is exposed due to the loss of enamel and/or soft tissue loss with gingival recession (including the loss of cementum). Once the dentin has been exposed, patent dentin tubules will be open to the oral environment, and lesion initiation occurs and as a consequence any subsequent stimuli may initiate minute fluid movement within the tubules, activating the mechanoreceptors in the inner third of the dentin. The loss of enamel due to abrasion and erosion may be a factor here, but acid erosion appears to be the predominant factor in DH. The presence of exposed dentin following these processes however does not always result in dentin hypersensitivity as occlusion of patent tubules may occur due to environmental desensitising mechanisms, the repair processes of secondary or sclerosed dentin or other naturally occurring factors (Orchardson and Gillam 2006).

It is however essential that the dental professional obtains an accurate history and conducts a thorough clinical examination (using the appropriate assessment) of the complaint in order to obtain a diagnosis of DH (including any associated aetiological or predisposing factors). This examination should also evaluate the impact of DH on the patient's quality of life. The dental professional would also be advised to undertake a stepwise approach when treating patients with DH which enables them to incorporate a preventive strategy aimed at removing any aetiological and predisposing factors in tandem with an initial non-invasive approach (Fig. 6.1). For example, the patient should be regularly reviewed for signs of attrition, abrasion, erosion and abfraction together with the appropriate dietary advice. Any change or correction of oral hygiene practices and incorrect or aggressive toothbrushing habits may also be considered at this time. A further factor to be considered is the timing of toothbrushing (before/after meals) as brushing following an acid challenge may lead to further loss of hard tissue (enamel, cementum). Patients may not however be able to remember in detail

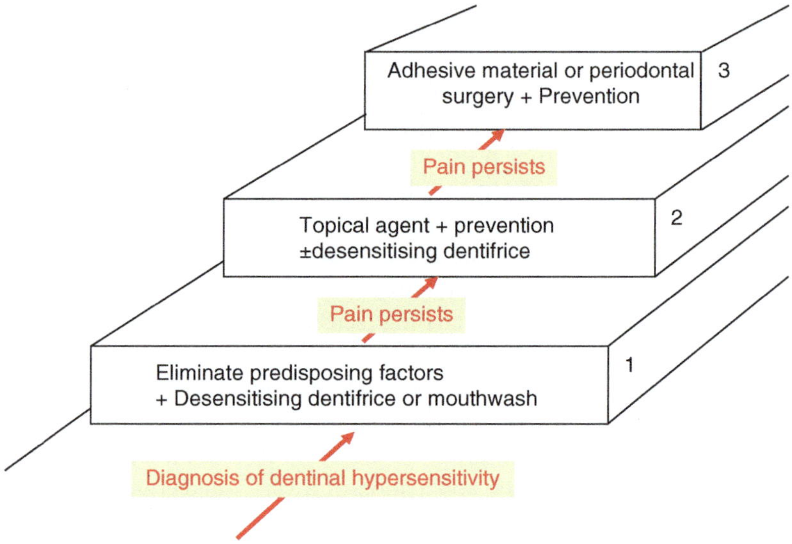

Fig. 6.1 A stepwise approach to treating dentin hypersensitivity (Acknowledgement Orchardson and Gillam (2006))

what they normally eat or drink, and the use of diet history sheets may also be of benefit. Any subsequent dietary advice should therefore be based on the analysis of these diet sheets prior to providing a personalised recommendation on the control of the consumption of acidic food and drink, commonly associated with DH (Addy et al. 1987), and on high sugar concentration products that provide the nutritional environment for root caries lesions. These carious lesions may also be restored by conventional restorative techniques, in situations where these lesions are not cleansable. The application of desensitising toothpastes and bonding agents, to occlude or seal the dentinal tubules, has been proposed for the treatment of DH, whereas high fluoride concentration varnishes and dentifrices (e.g. Duraphat) may also be used in treating both DH and root caries. If the initial treatment is unsuccessful, then the dental professional has the opportunity to try alternative strategies including a more invasive approach as indicated in Fig. 6.1. For example, it may be not only prudent but also economical for the dental professional to initiate treatment for a mild generalised sensitivity with an at-home product such as a desensitising toothpaste, and if this is not successful, then an in-office product or technique may be recommended. For patients with a localised moderate to severe sensitivity, the use of in-office products (primers, varnishes,sealants, glass ionomers, composite restorations) may be more appropriate. The dental professional should also be aware that in the more severe cases of dentin hypersensitivity, this stepwise approach may not necessarily resolve the patient's problem, and pulpal extirpation or extraction of the offending tooth (or teeth) may be the treatment of choice. It is also important for the dental professional to recognise that certain restorative procedures may contribute to dentin hypersensitivity, for example, the placement of sub-gingival restorations and crowns that may retain plaque or affect the biological width of the periodontal tissues. Alternative treatment modalities have also been recommended for the treatment of exposed dentin surface with associated dentin hypersensitivity, for example, the application of periodontal flap surgery (including Guided Tissue Regeneration [GTR], connective tissue grafts +/− Emdogain). It is therefore essential for the dental professional to review and monitor the problem on an appropriate basis and reassess if the pain persists. A number of management algorithms have been proposed that have incorporated a monitoring strategy for the management of DH (Addy and Urquhart 1992; Canadian Advisory Board on Dentin Hypersensitivity 2003; Orchardson and Gillam 2006; West 2007; Pashley et al. 2008) (Fig. 6.2).

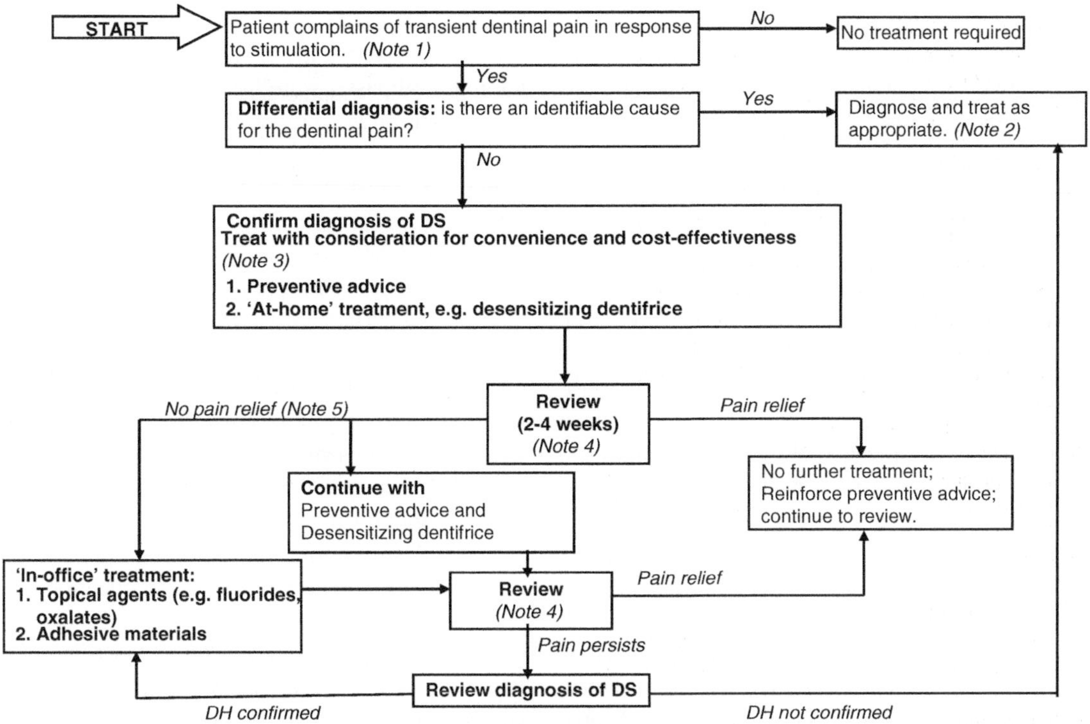

Fig. 6.2 Flowchart for the clinical management of dentin hypersensitivity (DH) (Orchardson and Gillam 2006) (Adapted with permission of George Warman Publications [UK] Ltd., from Addy and Urquhart (1992))
Note 1. Pain evoked by thermal, evaporative (jet of air), probe, osmotic or chemical stimuli
Note 2. Alternative causes of tooth pain include caries, chipped teeth, cracked tooth syndrome, fractured or leaking restorations, gingivitis, palatogingival grooves, postrestoration sensitivity or pulpitis
Note 3. Treatment may be delivered in a stratified manner, as indicated in Fig. 6.1. With localised or severe DH, practitioners may prefer to treat the patient directly, using an in-office procedure
Note 4. Some form of follow-up is recommended. However, the follow up interval may vary, depending on the patient's or practitioner's preference and circumstances
Note 5. If mild sensitivity persists at the initial follow-up appointment, the practitioner may continue with preventive and at-home therapies. If the sensitivity is more severe, some form of in-office treatment may be appropriate

6.3 At-Home Treatment Modalities

Following a clinical examination where the extent and severity of the problem is of a more generalised nature, with mild to moderate severity, a dental professional may recommend (to the patient) an at-home (or over-the-counter (OTC)) treatment rather than undertake any invasive dental procedures. As indicated above (Sect. 6.1) it is essential for the dental professional to consider implementing preventative strategies within the overall management of the problem. A number of 'at-home' products have been recommended by dental professionals to alleviate any discomfort from DH, and these have included toothpastes, mouthwash and gels; more recently the use of bleaching and whitening kits has included desensitising products such as potassium nitrate in order to reduce any associated dentin hypersensitivity. The prescription of toothpastes with a high fluoride concentration (2,800/5,000 ppm) (Duraphat) has also been recommended. The majority of 'at-home' products are, however, available in the form of OTC products for twice daily use by patients either in the form of a toothpaste or mouthwash. Historically strontium (chloride/acetate)-, stannous- or potassium (chloride, citrate, nitrate)-containing toothpastes have been marketed as desensitising toothpastes; more recently a number of other products such as casein phosphopeptide–amorphous calcium phosphate (CPP-ACP), bioactive glass, hydroxyapatite, propolis and calcium carbonate and arginine (Pro-Argin) have been developed in order to treat DH. Although these products appear to be commercially successful, the results from the published studies however would appear to show varying degrees of clinical efficacy for these products in clinical trials. There are problems however when analysing the results from these studies, and this is due in part to the differences in study design, methodology, study duration, variation in products over time [in different studies], reported placebo effects, etc. (Gillam and Newman 1993; Holland et al. 1997). For example, while there is some evidence for the efficacy of strontium-containing toothpastes (Markowitz 2009) either in a strontium chloride product (Carrasco 1971; Gedalia et al. 1978; Uchida et al. 1980; Minkoff and Axelrod 1987; Gillam et al. 1996a, b; Kobler et al. 2008) or a strontium acetate product (Pearce et al. 1994; Gillam et al. 1996a; West et al. 1997; Hughes et al. 2010; Mason et al. 2010), a number of reviews have been less favourable (Zappa 1994; Jackson 2000; Cummings 2009; Karim and Gillam 2013). According to Jackson (2000) none of the studies on strontium toothpastes demonstrated a consistent, significant improvement in the participants' symptoms from DH when compared with the negative control toothpaste. There also appears to be no supportive evidence from the published literature for strontium salts enhancing the deposition of the ingredients of the toothpaste or increasing the durability of the deposit on the tooth surface (Jackson 2000). A similar picture emerges when evaluating potassium-containing toothpastes despite the vast numbers of published studies (Tarbet et al. 1980, 1981; Silverman 1985; Silverman et al. 1994; Nagata et al. 1994; Salvato et al. 1992; Schiff et al. 1994, 1998, 2000; Sowinski et al. 2000, 2001; Wara-aswapati et al. 2005; Yates et al. 2005), and a number of investigators have raised concerns with regard to the efficacy of potassium-containing toothpastes which has led to the suggestion that potassium-containing toothpastes may be no more effective than regular fluoride toothpaste (Gillam et al. 1996a; West et al. 1997; Jackson 2000; Orchardson and Gillam 2000; Cummings 2009). The lack of data on the efficacy of potassium-containing toothpastes in reducing DH has also been highlighted in a number of systematic reviews (Poulsen et al. 2006; Pol et al. 2010; Karim and Gillam 2013). According to Karim and Gillam's (2013) recent review, there appears to be insufficient evidence to state categorically whether strontium or potassium salts per se are effective in reducing DH. There is also limited data on the efficacy of the other products used to treat dentin, for example, CPP-ACP toothpastes have been demonstrated to have a remineralising effect on enamel rather than a desensitising effect (Yengopal and Mickenautsch 2009; Azarpazhooh and Limeback 2008), although a recent study by Rosaiah and Aruna (2011) reported that multiple applications of G.C. tooth mousse and a single application of a Gluma Desensitizer had a more lasting desensitising effect when compared to ACP over 6 months. Bioactive glass (NovaMin®), hydroxyapatite and propolis toothpastes have also been reported to provide a desensitising effect (Du Min et al. 2008; Litkowski and Greenspan 2010; Sharma et al. 2010; Mahmoud et al. 1999; Madhavan et al. 2012; Ananthakrishna et al. 2012; Rajesh et al. 2012; Acharya et al. 2013). More recently Pro-Argin, a calcium carbonate and arginine complex based on Kleinberg's original formulation SensiStat (Kleinberg 2002), has been demonstrated to reduce DH in randomised clinical trials compared to either placebo or comparator products (Petrou et al. 2009; Ayad et al. 2009; Docimo et al. 2009; Elias Boneta et al. 2013a, b). Although conventional fluoride-containing toothpastes have been suggested as desensitising toothpastes, there is little evidence to support this claim (Gillam and Orchardson 2006; West 2007). Evidence from the published studies would suggest that these products are used as negative control toothpastes and generally speaking would not perform as well as recognised desensitising toothpastes. The question as to whether high concentration of fluoride in toothpastes such as 2,800/5,000 ppm (Duraphat) may be effective as desensitisers has not been fully explored although they have a recognised anticaries effect (Nordström and Birkhed 2010; Walsh et al. 2010).

Most of the published studies on these at-home products are generally of short duration of up to 12 weeks of product use in well-controlled studies using subjects that have a history of DH and respond to the methodology used to elicit a response. The question as to whether these subjects are truly representative of the normal population that have DH and routinely use a desensitising product has not been fully explored. Furthermore evidence from in vitro studies would appear to show that most of these products are susceptible to an acid challenge which may suggest that over time their ability to maintain a desensitising effect may be impaired. It is evident from the vast range of at-home products readily available for individuals complaining of DH that to date there is not an ideal desensitising product that fully satisfies Grossman's original criteria (or Gillam's modification) for an ideal desensitiser.

6.4 In-Office Treatment Modalities

A number of in-office treatment modalities for treating dentin hypersensitivity have been reported in the published literature (Pashley 2000; Orchardson and Gillam 2006; Lin et al. 2013). Pashley (2000) classified these in-office treatment modalities on the basis of (1) whether they do not polymerise (varnishes/precipitants/primers containing HEMA), (2) whether they undergo setting or polymerisation reactions (conventional glass ionomer cements, or resin-reinforced glass ionomers/compomers; adhesive resin primers; adhesive resin bonding systems), (3) the use of mouthguards, (4) iontophoresis and (5) lasers. According to Pashley (2000) most of these therapies have a degree of support of their efficacy for the treatment of DH (Table 6.1, 6.2, 6.3, 6.4, and 6.5). Generally speaking in-office treatment modalities involve patients who complain of DH localised to one or two teeth with moderate to severe discomfort and as such would require immediate attention. As with the management of DH using recommended at-home products, it is important that the dental professional incorporates a workable management and monitoring strategy based on preventive measures prior to offering a treatment option. Furthermore it is important to recognise that the patient may have DH from restorative procedures apart from those associated with loss of the hard tissue (e.g. non-carious cervical lesions). For example, the treatment of post-operative sensitivity may involve the application of a desensitiser underneath a crown or restoration (Haywood 2002; Jalandar et al. 2012) as well as post-operative sensitivity following periodontal therapy

Table 6.1 Summary of the published studies supporting the efficacy of in-office products (solutions and products)

Type, chemical/concentration	Product and clinical support
Fluorides	
Sodium fluoride, stannous fluoride, hydrogen fluoride	Dentinbloc, Colgate Oral Pharmaceuticals, Canton MA, USA (Thrash et al. 1992; Morris et al. 1999)
Nerve desensitisers	
Potassium nitrate	
1–15 % solutions	Hodosh (1974)
5 %, 10 % in gel	Frechoso et al. (2003)
Guanethidine monosulphate	
1 % guanethidine monosulphate	Ismelin, Ciba-Geigy (Dunne and Hannington-Kiff 1993)
Oxalate	
3 % potassium oxalate	Protect, Sunstar Butler, Chicago, IL, USA (Camps and Pashley 2003)
3 % potassium oxalate	Oxa-gel, Art-dent Ltda, Araraquara SP, Brazil (Pillon et al. 2004)
6.8 % ferric oxalate	Sensodyne Sealant, GSK, Jersey City NJ, USA (Gillam et al. 2004)
Calcium phosphates	
1.5M calcium chloride + 1.0M potassium oxalate	ACP-CPP, GC corporation, Tokyo, Japan (Geiger et al. 2003; Rosaiah and Aruna 2011)

Acknowledgement: Orchardson and Gillam (2006), Pashley et al. (2008) modified

Table 6.2 Summary of the published studies supporting the efficacy of in-office products (solutions and products)

Type, chemical/concentration	Product and clinical support
Desensitizing pastes	
Colgate® Sensitive Pro-Relief™ Desensitizing paste with 8 % arginine and calcium carbonate (Arg/$CaCO_3$)	Pro- Argin™ (Colgate Professional) (Hamlin et al. 2009; Schiff et al. 2009; Li et al. 2011)
elmex SENSITIVE Professional desensitizing paste	Pro- Argin™ Formulation GABA International Switzerland (Hamlin et al. 2012)
15 % calcium sodium phosphosilicate (CSPS; NovaMin(®)	Nupro® Sensodyne prophylaxis paste (Dentsply International) (Milleman et al. 2012; Neuhaus et al. 2013)
MI Paste Plus™ containing casein phosphopeptide–amorphous calcium phosphate (CCP-ACP) with 0.2 % sodium fluoride	(MI Paste Plus™ GC Corporation, www.gcamerica.com) According to the manufacturer both MI Paste and *MI Paste Plus* have FDA 510 K Clearance as a prophylaxis paste and for treating dentin hypersensitivity

Acknowledgement: Orchardson and Gillam (2006), Pashley et al. (2008) modified

Table 6.3 Summary of the published studies supporting the efficacy of in-office products (adhesives, resins and cements)

Type	Product and clinical support
Fluoride varnish	Duraphat, Colgate Oral Pharmaceuticals, Canton, MA, USA (Gaffar 1999; Corona et al. 2003; Merika et al. 2006)
	Fluoline, PD Dental, Altenwalde, Germany (Duran and Sengun 2004)
	Fluor Protector (Ivoclar Vivadent) (Ritter et al. 2006)
Oxalic acid + resin	MS Coat, Sun Medical Co, Shiga, Japan (Prati et al. 2001)
	Pain-Free, Parkell Co, Farmingdale, NY, USA (Morris et al. 1999)
Sealants, primers	Seal and Protect, Dentsply Konstanz, Germany (Baysan and Lynch 2003)
	Dentin Protector, Vivadent, Germany (Schwarz et al. 2002)
	Gluma Desensitizer, Heraeus Kulzer, Dormagen, Germany (Dondi dall'Orologio and Malferrari 1993; Duran and Sengun 2004; Dondi dall'Orologio et al. 1999, 2002; Kakaboura et al. 2005; Polderman and Frencken 2007)
	Gluma Alternate, Heraeus Kulzer, Wehrheim, Germany (Dondi dall'Orologio et al. 1999)
	Health-Dent Desensitizer, Healthdent Inc, Oswego, NY, USA (Duran and Sengun 2004; Dondi dall'Orologio et al. 1999)
	HEMA + other, HurriSeal Dentin Desensitizer Beutlich Pharmaceuticals LLC Waukegan, IL, USA, HemaSeal and Cide (Germiphene Corporation, Canada) (Kolker et al. 2002)
	Prime and Bond 2.1, Dentsply Caulk, Milford DE, USA (Swift et al. 2001)
	Scotchbond (Single Bond), 3M Dental Products, St Paul, MN, USA (Duran and Sengun 2004; Prati et al. 2001; Ferrari et al. 1999)
	One-Step Bisco Schaumburg IL, USA (Kakaboura et al. 2005)
Etch + primer	Scotchbond, 3M Dental Products, St Paul, MN, USA (Ferrari et al. 1999)
	Systemp.desensitizer, Ivoclar Vivadent, Schaan, Liechtenstein (Stewardson et al. 2004)
Etch + primer + adhesive	Scotchbond Multi-Purpose, 3M Dental Products, St Paul MN, USA (Dondi dall'Orologio et al. 1999, 2002)
Primer + adhesive	SE Bond, Kuraray, Okayama, Japan (Duran and Sengun 2004)
Glass ionomer cements/ resin-reinforced glass ionomer	Vitrebond-like (3M-ESPE, St. Paul, Minnesota USA), Fuji VI1 (GC Asia Dental Pte Ltd, Singapore, Hansen 1992; Tantbirojn et al. 2006; Polderman and Frencken 2007)

Acknowledgement: Orchardson and Gillam (2006), Pashley et al. (2008) modified

(von Troil et al. 2003, Gillam and Orchardson 2006; Lin and Gillam 2012). Dentin hypersensitivity arising from periodontal therapy, for example, scaling procedures, may be initially alleviated in the clinical setting by the application of desensitising polishing pastes such as Pro-Argin™ (Colgate Professional) or NovaMin products (Nupro® Sensodyne prophylaxis paste Dentsply

Table 6.4 Summary of the published studies supporting the efficacy of miscellaneous in-office techniques

Technique and clinical support	
Iontophoresis	Gangarosa and Park (1978), Brough et al. (1985), Gupta et al. (2010), Aparna et al. (2010)
Hypnosis/hypnotherapy	Starr et al. (1989), Eitner et al. (2010)
Laser therapy	Renton-Harper and Midda (1992), Kimura et al. (2000), Yilmaz et al. (2011a, b), Umberto et al. (2012)

Table 6.5 Summary of the published studies supporting the efficacy of at-home products

Product and clinical support	
10 % strontium chloride toothpaste (no fluoride)	Carrasco (1971), Gedalia et al. (1978), Uchida et al. (1980), Minkoff and Axelrod (1987), Gillam et al. (1992a, b), Kobler et al. (2008), Kumar et al. (2010)
8 % strontium acetate and 1,050 ppm fluoride	Pearce et al. (1994), Gillam et al. (1996a), West et al. (1997), Hughes et al. (2010), Mason et al. (2010)
2–5 % potassium-containing toothpastes in the form of nitrate, chloride or citrate	Tarbet et al. (1980, 1981), Silverman (1985) Silverman et al. (1996, 1994), Nagata et al. (1994), Salvato et al. (1992), Schiff et al. (1994, 1998, 2000), Sowinski et al. (2000, 2001), Wara-aswapati et al. (2005), Yates et al. (2005), Barlow et al. (2012)
3 % potassium-containing mouthwash	Gillam et al. (1996b), Yates et al. (1998), Pereira and Chava (2001)
Pro-Argin toothpastes containing 80,000 ppm (8 %) arginine, bicarbonate and calcium carbonate and 1,450 ppm fluorine as NaMFP (also elmex SENSITIVE)	Nathoo et al. (2009), Petrou et al. (2009), Ayad et al. (2009), Docimo et al. (2009), Que et al. (2010), Kakar et al. (2012), Elias Boneta et al. (2013a)
Pro-Argin mouthwash containing 0.8 % arginine, pyrophosphate and PVM/MA copolymer	Hu et al. (2013), Elias Boneta et al. (2013a, b)
Calcium sodium phosphosilicate (NovaMin®), 1,450 ppm fluoride	Du Min et al. (2008), Litkowski and Greenspan (2010), Sharma et al. (2010), Ananthakrishna et al. (2012), Rajesh et al. (2012), Acharya et al. (2013)
Tooth mousse MI Plus casein phosphopeptide amorphous calcium phosphate (CPP-ACP), 900 ppm fluoride	Geiger et al. (2003), Rosaiah and Aruna (2011), Madhavan et al. (2012)
elmex® SENSITIVE PLUS toothpaste containing amine fluoride (1,400 ppm F)	Renggli (1997)
elmex SENSITIVE mouthwash containing 250 ppm F (125 ppm F from amine fluoride, 125 ppm F from potassium fluoride	Zappa (1999)
Propolis	Mahmoud et al. (1999), Madhavan et al. (2012)
Hydroxyapatite toothpaste	Kang et al. (2009), Shetty et al. (2010), Orsini et al. (2010)

International) prior to the provision of an OTC desensitising toothpaste for home use (Hamlin et al. 2009; Schiff et al. 2009; Milleman et al. 2012; Neuhaus et al. 2013). The use of desensitising products in bleaching gels may also help alleviate bleaching sensitivity particularly in patients with or without pre-existing DH (Haywood 2002). A number of investigators have also utilised various gingival grafting techniques in order to treat marginal gingival defects and/or correct aesthetic concerns (Gillam and Orchardson 2006). The majority of these published studies however deal with specific surgical techniques and materials designed to alleviate the clinical outcomes of gingival recession rather than evaluating DH per se. According to Gillam and Orchardson (2006), the reported prevalence of DH following the surgical procedures is 17–30 %, and the associated discomfort lasts approximately 4–6 weeks. A recent review by Douglas de Oliveira et al. (2013) however suggested that there was insufficient clinical evidence to conclude that surgical root coverage procedures predictably reduce DH although the procedures may reduce DH and have a positive impact on a patient's quality of life (de Oliveira et al. 2013).

Several investigators (Starr et al. 1989; Eitner et al. 2010) have also evaluated the use of hypnosis or hypnotherapy in the treatment of DH. The study by Starr et al. involved only 8 patients, and while all patients demonstrated significant improvements in symptoms following hypnosis, these investigators did not use any recognisable DH methodology to evaluate the pain response. The study by Eitner et al. (2010) involving a larger sample of 102 patients attempted to compare recognised desensitising therapies (fluoride [elmex gelee and elmex SENSITIVE toothpaste], Gluma Desensitizer) with hypnotherapy using Visual Analogue Scales (VAS) and response to a cold stimulus in a 1-month study. These investigators reported that although no statistically significant differences were observed between the three groups, there was a noticeable difference with regard to both the onset and duration of the observed effect of the desensitiser and hypnosis groups compared to the fluoride group. This observation may however be explained on the basis of the different mode of action of an in-office desensitiser and a medical intervention compared to an at-home fluoride toothpaste as well as associated placebo and non-placebo effects. It was not clear from the study whether the non-fluoride groups used different toothpastes as part of their normal oral hygiene regimen. Nevertheless hypnotherapy may be an option for some patients with DH although as Eitner et al. concluded, more studies are needed in order to validate the results from this study.

There have been a number of reviews that have investigated the vast array of products and procedures that dental professionals have used to treat DH, and it is evident that there is no widespread agreement as to which is the best material or procedure to treat DH (Gillam 1992; Orchardson and Gillam 2006; Cunha-Cruz et al. 2010; Lin et al. 2013). This is due in part to the highly subjective nature of the pain response as well as the differing methodologies used to evaluate the various desensitising agents or techniques. For example, several investigators have recommended the use and application of fluoride with or without iontophoresis (Gangarosa and Park 1978; Brough et al. 1985; Gupta et al. 2010; Aparna et al. 2010) although the clinical efficacy of this technique has been questioned (Gillam and Newman 1990; Pashley 2000). The use of laser technology has also been advocated for the treatment of dentin hypersensitivity (Renton-Harper and Midda 1992; Kimura et al. 2000; Yilmaz et al. 2011a, b; Umberto et al. 2012), and a number of studies have reported a degree of efficacy for this therapy (He et al. 2011) although as West (2007) indicated the clinical results from these studies are somewhat equivocal in nature. There are however a number of problems when evaluating the results from these studies, for example, most of these studies have relatively small sample sizes and different control groups as well as different laser systems such as a neodymium-doped yttrium, aluminium, garnet (Nd:YAG); erbium, chromium:yttrium, scandium, gallium (Er:YSG); erbium, chromium-doped:yttrium, scandium, gallium, garnet (Er,Cr:YSGG); carbon dioxide (CO2); and diode which make analysis of the results difficult to interpret. Furthermore, the laser treatment may not be blinded from the subject, and it could also be practically challenging for the dental professional to produce uniform laser treatment of irregular-shaped lesions using a hand-held light guide especially if the laser operates in a pulsing mode (Pashley 2000). Associated placebo effects may also be interfering with the true extent of the efficacy of this technique, and more studies with larger sample sizes should be undertaken before this technique can be recognised as an acceptable treatment for treating DH (West 2007). The recent systematic review by He et al. (2011) reported that laser therapy had a slight clinical advantage over topical desensitising products such as fluoride varnishes although Lier et al. (2002) reported that the effect of treating sensitive teeth with a Nd:YAG laser was no different from the placebo control. Although laser therapy appears to be an area of interest from a research viewpoint, there seems to be a limited use of lasers in dental practice when treating dentin sensitivity. For example, Cunha-Cruz et al. (2010) reported that laser therapy was rarely used and considered relatively unsuccessful by a sample of 209 American dentists when asked to report on which treatments they would use when treating DH. A number of recent systematic reviews have also evaluated the reported efficacy of in-office products recommended for the treatment of dentin hypersensitivity (Cunha-Cruz et al. 2011; He et al. 2011; Lin et al. 2013). It was also apparent from the study by Cunha-Cruz et al. (2010) that dental professionals not only appear to be uncertain as to the most successful way in which to manage DH but also express a level of dissatisfaction with the various products and techniques available. These reviews would therefore appear to confirm that there is no currently agreed gold standard for treating DH although most products and techniques appear to have a degree of success when treating the condition.

Conclusions

From reviewing the available literature on the condition, it is apparent that the availability of a vast array of treatment modalities would indicate either that there is no one effective desensitising agent for completely resolving the discomfort or that the condition due to its highly subjective nature is difficult to treat irrespective of the available treatment options. There are problems however in evaluating the efficacy of both at-home and in-office treatment modalities due to the variation in the study design, methodology of assessment, relatively small sample size, changes in formulations over time, influence of placebo effects and duration of the publishing studies. For the dental professional to successfully manage DH and to enable their patients to have an improved quality of life, it is essential not only to correctly diagnose the condition but also to initiate a simple yet practical management strategy. This should be based on a stepwise approach, incorporating preventative and management strategies, in order to identify and eliminate any predisposing factors, in particular erosive factors (e.g. dietary acids) prior to offering any treatment to the patient. Treatment should be subsequently based on the extent and severity of the problem, for example, if the patient has severe discomfort limited to one or two teeth, then an in-office procedure would be the first treatment option of choice. If the patient's discomfort is initially of a generalised mild disposition, then it would be appropriate for an at-home product to be provided; however, if the discomfort is not resolved by this method after a few weeks, then it would be appropriate for the dental professional to re-examine the patient and treat as necessary with an in-office procedure. It would be prudent for the dental professional to recognise that there is no one ideal treatment modality when treating DH and there may be occasions when a combination of at-home and in-office treatment may be appropriate to resolve the problem and provide the patient with an improvement in their quality of life.

References

Acharya AB, Surve SM, Thakur SL (2013) A clinical study of the effect of calcium sodium phosphosilicate on dentin hypersensitivity. J Clin Exp Dent 5(1):e18–22

Addy M, Urquhart E (1992) Dentine hypersensitivity: Its prevalence, aetiology and clinical management. Dent 19(10):407–8, 410–2

Addy M, Mostafa P, Newcombe R (1987) Dentine hypersensitivity. A comparison of five toothpastes used during a 6-week treatment period. Br Dent J 163:45–50

Ananthakrishna S, Raghu TN, Koshy S, Kumar N (2012) Clinical evaluation of the efficacy of bioactive glass and strontium chloride for treatment of dentinal hypersensitivity. J Interdiscip Dentistry 2:92–7

Aparna S, Setty S, Thakur S (2010) Comparative efficacy of two treatment modalities for dentinal hypersensitivity: a clinical trial. Indian J Dent Res 21(4):544–8. doi:10.4103/0970-9290.74213

Ayad F, Ayad N, Zhang YP, DeVizio W, Cummins D, Mateo LR (2009) Comparing the efficacy in reducing dentin hypersensitivity of a new toothpaste containing 8.0% arginine, calcium carbonate, and 1450 ppm fluoride to a commercial sensitive toothpaste containing 2% potassium ion: An eight week clinical study on Canadian adults. J Clin Dent 20(Spec Iss):10–16

Azarpazhooh A, Limeback H (2008) Clinical efficacy of casein derivatives: a systematic review of the literature. J Am Dent Assoc 139(7):915–924

Barlow AP, He J, Tian C, Jeffery P, Mason SC, Tai BJ, Jiang H, Rees GD, Du MQ (2012) A comparative evaluation of the efficacy of two novel desensitising dentifrices. Int J Dent 2012:896143. doi:10.1155/2012/896143, Epub 2012 Dec 6

Baysan A, Lynch E (2003) Treatment of cervical sensitivity with a root sealant. Am J Dent 16(2):135–8
Bekes K, John MT, Schaller HG, Hirsch C (2009) Oral health-related quality of life in patients seeking care for dentin hypersensitivity. J Oral Rehabil 36(1):45–51
Brough KM, Anderson DM, Love J, Overman PR (1985) The effectiveness of iontophoresis in reducing dentin hypersensitivity. J Am Dent Assoc 111(5):761–5
Camps J, Pashley D (2003) In vivo sensitivity of human root dentin to air blast and scratching. J Periodontol 74(11):1589–94
Canadian Advisory Board on Dentin Hypersensitivity (2003) Consensus-based recommendations for the diagnosis and management of dentin hypersensitivity. J Can Dent Assoc 69(4):221–6
Carrasco HP (1971) Strontium chloride toothpaste–effectiveness as related to duration of use. Pharmacol Ther Dent 1(4):209–15
Corona SA, Nascimento TN, Catirse AB, Lizarelli RF, Dinelli W, Palma-Dibb RG (2003) Clinical evaluation of low-level laser therapy and fluoride varnish for treating cervical dentinal hypersensitivity. J Oral Rehabil 30(12):1183–9
Cummins D (2009) Dentin hypersensitivity: from diagnosis to a breakthrough therapy for everyday sensitivity relief. J Clin Dent 20(1):1–9, Review
Cummins D (2010) Recent advances in dentin hypersensitivity: clinically proven treatments for instant and lasting sensitivity. Am J Dent 23(Special Issue A): 1A–13A
Cunha-Cruz J, Wataha JC, Zhou L, Manning W, Trantow M, Bettendorf MM, Heaton LJ, Berg J (2010) Treating dentin hypersensitivity: therapeutic choices made by dentists of the northwest PRECEDENT network. J Am Dent Assoc 141(9):1097–105
Cunha-Cruz J, Stout JR, Heaton LJ, Wataha JC (2011) Dentin hypersensitivity and oxalates: a systematic review. J Dent Res 90(3):304–10
Dababneh RH, Khouri AT, Addy M (1999) Dentine hypersensitivity – an enigma? A review of terminology, epidemiology, mechanisms, aetiology and management. Br Dent J 187(11):606–11
de Oliveira DW, Marques DP, Aguiar-Cantuária IC, Flecha OD, Gonçalves PF (2013) Effect of surgical defect coverage on cervical dentin hypersensitivity and quality of life. J Periodontol; 84(6):768–75. doi: 10.1902/jop.2012.120479 [Epub 2012 Aug 16]
Douglas de Oliveira DW, Oliveira-Ferreira F, Flecha OD, Gonçalves PF (2013) Is surgical root coverage effective for the treatment of cervical dentin hypersensitivity? A systematic review. J Periodontol 84(3):295–306. doi:10.1902/jop.2012.120143, Epub 2012 May
Docimo R, Montesani L, Maturo P, Costacurta M, Bartolino M, DeVizio W, Zhang YP, Cummins D, Dibart S, Mateo LR (2009) Comparing the efficacy in reducing dentin hypersensitivity of a new toothpaste containing 8.0%arginine, calcium carbonate, and 1450 ppm fluoride to a commercial sensitive toothpaste containing 2% potassium ion: an eight-week clinical study in Rome, Italy. J Clin Dent 20(Spec Iss):17–22
Dondi dall'Orologio G, Malferrari S (1993) Desensitizing effects of Gluma and Gluma 2000 on hypersensitive dentin. Am J Dent 6(6):283–6
Dondi dall'Orologio G, Lorenzi R, Anselmi M, Opisso V (1999) Dentin desensitizing effects of Gluma Alternate, Health-Dent Desensitizer and Scotchbond Multi-Purpose. Am J Dent 12(3):103–6
Dondi dall'Orologio G, Lone A, Finger WJ (2002) Clinical evaluation of the role of glutardialdehyde in a one-bottle adhesive. Am J Dent. 15(5):330–4
Drisko CH (2002) Dentin hypersensitivity—dental hygiene and periodontal considerations. Int Dent J 52:385–393
Du Min Q, Bian Z, Jiang H, Greenspan DC, Burwell AK, Zhong J, Tai BJ (2008) Clinical evaluation of a dentifrice containing calcium sodium phosphosilicate (novamin) for the treatment of dentin hypersensitivity. Am J Dent 21(4):210–4
Dunne SM, Hannington-Kiff JG (1993) The use of topical guanethidine in the relief of dentine hypersensitivity: a controlled study. Pain 54(2):165–8
Duran I, Sengun A (2004) The long-term effectiveness of five current desensitizing products on cervical dentine sensitivity. J Oral Rehabil 31(4):351–6
Eitner S, Bittner C, Wichmann M, Nickenig HJ, Sokol B (2010) Comparison of conventional therapies for dentin hypersensitivity versus medical hypnosis. Int J Clin Exp Hypn 58(4):457–75
Elias Boneta AR, Ramirez K, Naboa J, Mateo LR, Stewart B, Panagokos F, De Vizio W (2013a) Efficacy in reducing dentine hypersensitivity of a regimen using a toothpaste containing 8 % arginine and calcium carbonate, a mouthwash containing 0.8 % arginine, pyrophosphate and PVM/MA copolymer and a toothbrush compared to potassium and negative control regimens: an eight-week randomized clinical trial. J Dent 41:s42–s49
Elias Boneta AR, Galán Salás RM, Mateo LR, Stewart B, Mello S, Arvanitidou LS, Panagakos F, DeVizio W (2013b) Efficacy of a mouthwash containing 0.8 % arginine, PVM/MA copolymer, pyrophosphates, and 0.05 % sodium fluoride compared to a commercial mouthwash containing 2.4 % potassium nitrate and 0.022 % sodium fluoride and a control mouthwash containing 0.05 % sodium fluoride on dentine hypersensitivity: a six-week randomized clinical study. J Dent Suppl 1:S34-41. doi: 10.1016/j.jdent.2012.11.004. [Epub 2013 Feb 1]
Ferrari M, Cagidiaco MC, Kugel G, Davidson CL (1999) Clinical evaluation of a one-bottle bonding system for desensitizing exposed roots. Am J Dent 12(5):243–9
Frechoso SC, Menéndez M, Guisasola C, Arregui I, Tejerina JM, Sicilia A (2003) Evaluation of the efficacy of two potassium nitrate bioadhesive gels (5% and 10%) in the treatment of dentine hypersensitivity. A randomised clinical trial. J Clin Periodontol 30(4): 315–20
Gaffar A (1999) Treating hypersensitivity with fluoride varnish. Compend Contin Educ Dent 20(1 Suppl): 27–33

Gangarosa LP, Park NH (1978) Practical considerations in iontophoresis of fluoride for desensitizing dentin. J Prosthet Dent 39(2):173–8

Gedalia I, Brayer L, Kalter N, Richter M, Stabholz A (1978) The effect of fluoride and strontium application on dentin: in vivo and in vitro studies. J Periodontol 49(5):269–72

Geiger S, Matalon S, Blasbalg J, Tung MS, Eichmiller FC (2003) The clinical effect of amorphous calcium phosphate (ACP) on root surface hypersensitivity. Oper Dent 28:496–500

Gibson B, Boiko OV, Baker S et al (2010) The everyday impact of dentine sensitivity: personal and functional aspects. Soc Sci Dent 1:11–20

Gillam DG (1992) The assessment and treatment of cervical dentinal sensitivity. DDS Thesis, University of Edinburgh, Scotland

Gillam DG (1997) Clinical trial designs for testing of products for dentine hypersensitivity–a review. J West Soc Periodontol Periodontal Abstr 45(2):37–46, Review

Gillam DG, Newman HN (1990) Iontophoresis in the treatment of cervical dentinal sensitivity–a review. J West Soc Periodontol Periodontal Abstr 38(4): 129–33

Gillam DG, Newman HN (1993) Assessment of pain in cervical dentinal sensitivity studies. A review. J Clin Periodontol 20(6):383–94

Gillam DG, Orchardson R (2006) Advances in the treatment of root dentine sensitivity: mechanisms and treatment principles. Endod Topics 13:13–33

Gillam DG, Turner W (2013) The management of gingival recession. Chapter 3.2 In: Textbook of Periodontics Eaton KE, Ower P (eds). Churchill Livingston; Elsevier Ltd (in press)

Gillam DG, Newman HN, Davies EH, Bulman JS (1992a) Clinical efficacy of a low abrasive dentifrice for the relief of cervical dentinal hypersensitivity. J Clin Periodontol 19:197–201

Gillam DG, Newman HN, Bulman JS, Davies EH (1992b) Dentifrice abrasivity and cervical dentinal hypersensitivity. Results 12 weeks following cessation of 8 weeks' supervised use. J Periodontol 63:7–12

Gillam DG, Bulman JS, Jackson RJ, Newman HN (1996a) Comparison of 2 desensitizing dentifrices with a commercially available fluoride dentifrice in alleviating cervical dentine sensitivity. J Periodontol 67(8): 737–42

Gillam DG, Bulman JS, Jackson RJ, Newman HN (1996b) Efficacy of a potassium nitrate mouthwash in alleviating cervical dentine sensitivity (CDS). J Clin Periodontol 23(11):993–7

Gillam DG, Newman HN, Davies EH, Bulman JS, Troullos ES, Curro FA (2004) Clinical evaluation of ferric oxalate in relieving dentine hypersensitivity. J Oral Rehabil 31(3):245–50

Grossman LI (1935) A systematic method for the treatment of hypersensitive dentine. J Am Dent Assoc 22:592–602

Gupta M, Pandit IK, Srivastava N, Gugnani N (2010) Comparative evaluation of 2% sodium fluoride iontophoresis and other cavity liners beneath silver amalgam restorations. J Indian Soc Pedod Prev Dent 28(2):68–72

Hamlin D, Williams KP, Delgado E, Zhang YP, DeVizio W, Mateo LR (2009) Clinical evaluation of the efficacy of a desensitizing paste containing 8% arginine and calcium carbonate for the in-office relief of dentin hypersensitivity associated with dental prophylaxis. Am J Dent 22(Sp Is A):16A–20A

Hamlin D, Mateo LR, Dibart S, Delgado E, Zhang YP, DeVizio W (2012) Comparative efficacy of two treatment regimens combining in-office and at-home programs for dentin hypersensitivity relief: a 24-week clinical study. Am J Dent. 25(3):146–52

Hansen EK (1992) Dentin hypersensitivity treated with a fluoride-containing varnish or a light-cured glass-ionomer liner. Eur J Oral Sci 100:305–309

Haywood VB (2002) Dentine hypersensitivity: bleaching and restorative considerations for successful management. Int Dent J 52:7–10

He S, Wang Y, Li X, Hu D (2011) Effectiveness of laser therapy and topical desensitising agents in treating dentine hypersensitivity: a systematic review. J Oral Rehabil 38(5):348–58

Hodosh M (1974) A superior desensitiser-potassium nitrate. J Am Dent Assoc 88:831–832

Holland GR, Narhi MN, Addy M, Gangarosa L, Orchardson R (1997) Guidelines for the design and conduct of clinical trials on dentine hypersensitivity. J Clin Periodontol 24(11):808–13

Hu D, Stewart B, Mello S, Arvanitidou L, Panagakos F, De Vizio W, Zhang YP, Mateo LR, Yin W (2013) Efficacy of a mouthwash containing 0.8 % arginine, PVM/MA copolymer, pyrophosphates, and 0.05 % sodium fluoride compared to a negative control mouthwash on dentin hypersensitivity reduction. A randomized clinical trial. J Dent. 41 Suppl 1:S26–33. doi: 10.1016/j.jdent.2012.10.001 [Epub 2013 Feb 1]

Hughes N, Mason S, Jeffery P, Welton H, Tobin M, O'Shea C, Browne M (2010) A comparative clinical study investigating the efficacy of a test dentifrice containing 8% strontium acetate and 1040 ppm sodium fluoride versus a marketed control dentifrice containing 8% arginine, calcium carbonate, and 1450 ppm sodium monofluorophosphate in reducing dentinal hypersensitivity. J Clin Dent 21(2):49–55

Jackson RJ (2000) Potential treatment modalities for dentine hypersensitivity: home use products. In: Addy M, Embery G, Edgar WM, Orchardson R (eds) Tooth wear sensitivity. Martin Dunitz, London, pp 328–338

Jalandar SS, Pandharinath DS, Arun K, Smita V (2012) Comparison of effect of desensitizing agents on the retention of crowns cemented with luting agents: an in vitro study. J Adv Prosthodont 4(3):127–33

Kakaboura A, Rahiotis C, Thomaidis S, Doukoudakis S (2005) Clinical effectiveness of two agents on the treatment of tooth cervical hypersensitivity. Am J Dent 18(4):291–5

Kakar A, Kakar K, Sreenivasan PK, DeVizio W, Kohli R (2012) Comparison of the clinical efficacy of a new dentifrice containing 8.0% arginine, calcium carbonate, and 1000 ppm fluoride to a commercially available sensitive toothpaste containing 2% potassium ion on dentin hypersensitivity: a randomized clinical trial. J Clin Dent 23(2):40–7

Kang S-J, Kwon Y-H, Park J-B, Herr Y, Chung J-H (2009) The effects of hydroxyapatite toothpaste on tooth hypersensitivity. J Korean Acad Periodontol 39(1):9–16

Karim BF, Gillam DG (2013) The efficacy of strontium and potassium toothpastes in treating dentine hypersensitivity: a systematic review. Int J Dent. 2013:573258. doi: 10.1155/2013/573258 [Epub 2013 Apr 8]

Kimura YP, Wilder-Smith K, Yonaga K, Matsumoto K (2000) Treatment of dentine hypersensitivity by lasers: a review. J Clin Periodontol 27:715–721

Kleinberg I (2002) SensiStat, a new saliva-based composition for simple and effective treatment of dentinal sensitivity pain. Dent Today 21:42–47

Kobler A, Kub O, Schaller H, Gernhardt CR (2008) Clinical effectiveness of a strontium chloride-containing desensitizing agent over 6 months: a randomized, double-blind, placebo-controlled study. Quintessence Int 39:321–325

Kolker JL, Vargas MA, Armstrong SR, Dawson DV (2002) Effect of desensitizing agents on dentin permeability and dentin tubule occlusion. J Adhes Dent 4(3):211–21

Kumar RV, Shubhashini N, Sheshan H, Kranti K (2010) A clinical trial comparing a stannous fluoride based dentifrice and a strontium chloride based dentifrice in alleviating dentinal hypersensitivity. J Int Oral Health 2:37–50

Li R, Tang XJ, Li YH, Wang Y, Chen J, Wang QH, Huang YJ, Zhou Z (2011) Arginine-containing desensitizing toothpaste for dentine hypersensitivity: a meta-analysis. Chinese Journal of Evidence-Based Medicine 11(5):570–575

Lier BB, Rösing CK, Aass AM, Gjermo P (2002) Treatment of dentin hypersensitivity by Nd:YAG laser. J Clin Periodontol 29(6):501–6

Lin YH, Gillam DG (2012) The prevalence of root sensitivity following periodontal therapy: a systematic review. Int J Dent 2012:407023. doi:10.1155/2012/407023, Epub 2012 Oct 31

Lin PY, Cheng YW, Chu CY, Chien KL, Lin CP, Tu YK (2013) In-office treatment for dentin hypersensitivity: a systematic review and network meta-analysis. J Clin Periodontol 40(1):53–64

Litkowski L, Greenspan DC (2010) A clinical study of the effect of calcium sodium phosphosilicate on dentin hypersensitivity–proof of principle. J Clin Dent 21(3):77–81

Madhavan S, Nayak M, Shenoy A, Shetty R, Prasad K (2012) Dentinal hypersensitivity: a comparative clinical evaluation of CPP-ACP F, sodium fluoride, propolis, and placebo. J Conserv Dent 15:315–8

Mahmoud AS, Almas K, Dahlan AA (1999) The effect of propolis on dentinal hypersensitivity and level of satisfaction among patients from a university hospital Riyadh, Saudi Arabia. Indian J Dent Res 10(4):130–7

Markowitz K (2009) The original desensitizers: strontium and potassium salts. J Clin Dent 20(5):145–51

Mason S, Hughes N, Sufi F, Bannon L, Maggio B, North M, Holt J (2010) A comparative clinical study investigating the efficacy of a dentifrice containing 8% strontium acetate and 1040 ppm fluoride in a silica base and a control dentifrice containing 1450 ppm fluoride in a silica base to provide immediate relief of dentin hypersensitivity. J Clin Dent 21(2):42–8

Merika K, HeftitArthur F, Preshaw PM (2006) Comparison of two topical treatments for dentine sensitivity. Eur J Prosthodont Restor Dent 14(1):38–41

Milleman JL, Milleman KR, Clark CE, Mongiello KA, Simonton TC, Proskin HM (2012) NUPRO sensodyne prophylaxis paste with NovaMin for the treatment of dentin hypersensitivity: a 4-week clinical study. Am J Dent 25(5):262–8

Minkoff S, Axelrod S (1987) Efficacy of strontium chloride in dental hypersensitivity. J Periodontol 58:470–74

Morris MF, Davis RD, Richardson BW (1999) Clinical efficacy of two dentin desensitizing agents. Am J Dent 12(2):72–6

Nagata T, Ishida H, Shinohara H, Kasahara S, Wakano Y, Daigen S, Troullos ES (1994) Clinical evaluation of a potassium nitrate dentifrice for the treatment of dentinal hypersensitivity. J Clin Periodontol 21:217–221

Nathoo S, Delgado E, Zhang YP, DeVizio W, Cummins D, Mateo LR (2009) Comparing the efficacy in providing instant relief of dentin hypersensitivity of a new toothpaste containing 8.0% arginine, calcium carbonate, and 1450 ppm fluoride relative to a benchmark desensitizing toothpaste containing 2% potassium ion and 1450 ppm fluoride, and to a control toothpaste with 1450 ppm fluoride: a three-day clinical study in New Jersey, USA. J Clin Dent 20(4):123–30

Neuhaus KW, Milleman JL, Milleman KR, Mongiello KA, Simonton TC, Clark CE, Proskin HM, Seemann R (2013) Effectiveness of a calcium sodium phosphosilicate containing prophylaxis paste in reducing dentine hypersensitivity immediately and 4 weeks after a single application: a double-blind randomized controlled trial. J Clin Periodontol 40(4):349–357

Nordström A, Birkhed D (2010) Preventive effect of high-fluoride dentifrice (5,000 ppm) in caries-active adolescents: a 2-year clinical trial. Caries Res 44(3):323–31

Ong G (1986) Desensitizing agents. A review. Clin Prev Dent 8(3):14–8

Orchardson R, Gillam DG (2000) The efficacy of potassium salts as agents for treating dentin hypersensitivity. J Orofac Pain 14:9–19

Orchardson R, Gillam DG (2006) Managing dentin hypersensitivity. J Am Dent Assoc 137(7):990–8

Orsini G, Procaccini M, Manzoli L, Giuliodori F, Lorenzini A, Putignano A (2010) A double-blind randomized-controlled trial comparing the desensitizing efficacy of a new dentifrice containing carbonate/hydroxyapatite nanocrystals and a sodium fluoride/potassium nitrate dentifrice. J Clin Periodontol 37(6):510–7

Pashley DH (2000) Potential treatment modalities for dentine hypersensitivity: in office products. In:

Addy M, Embery G, Edgar WM, Orchardson R (eds) Tooth wear and sensitivity. Martin Dunitz, London, pp 351–365

Pashley DH, Tay FR, Haywood VB, Collins MA, Drisko CL (2008) Consensus-based recommendations for the diagnosis and management of dentin hypersensitivity 4(9 Special Issue) Supplement to Inside Dentistry®

Pearce NX, Addy M, Newcombe RG (1994) Dentine hypersensitivity: a clinical trial to compare 2 strontium densensitizing toothpastes with a conventional fluoride toothpaste. J Periodontol 65(2):113–9

Pereira R, Chava VK (2001) Efficacy of a 3% potassium nitrate desensitizing mouthwash in the treatment of dentinal hypersensitivity. J Periodontol 72(12): 1720–5

Petrou I, Heu R, Stranick M, Lavender S, Zaidel L, Cummins D, Sullivan RJ, Hsueh C, Gimzewski JK (2009) A breakthrough therapy for dentin hypersensitivity: how dental products containing 8% arginine and calcium carbonate work to deliver effective relief of sensitive teeth. J Clin Dent 20(Spec Iss): 23–31

Pillon FL, Romani IG, Schmidt ER (2004) Effect of a 3% potassium oxalate topical application on dentinal hypersensitivity after subgingival scaling and root planing. J Periodontol 75:1461–1464

Pol DG, Jonnala J, Chute M, Gunjikar T, Pol S (2010) Desensitising agents "what is more preferable dentifrice or mouthwash?". J Indian Dent Assoc 4(22):486–487

Polderman RN, Frencken JE (2007) Comparison between effectiveness of a low-viscosity glass ionomer and a resin-based glutaraldehyde containing primer in treating dentine hypersensitivity–a 25.2-month evaluation. J Dent 35(2):144–9

Poulsen S, Errboe M, Lescay Mevil Y, Glenny AM (2006) Potassium containing toothpastes for dentine hypersensitivity. Cochrane Database Syst Rev 19(3):CD001476. Review

Prati C, Cervellati F, Sanasi V, Montebugnoli L (2001) Treatment of cervical dentin hypersensitivity with resin adhesives: 4-week evaluation. Am J Dent 14(6):378–82

Que K, Fu Y, Lin L, Hu D, Zhang YP, Panagakos FS et al (2010) Dentin hypersensitivity reduction of new toothpaste containing 8.0% arginine and 1450 ppm fluoride: an 8-week clinical study on Chinese adults. Am J Dent 23A(Special Issue):28A–35A

Rajesh KS, Hedge S, Arun Kumar MS, Shetty DG (2012) Evaluation of the efficacy of a 5% calcium sodium phosphosilicate (Novamin®) containing dentifrice for the relief of dentinal hypersensitivity: a clinical study. Indian J Dent Res 23:363–7

Renggli HH (1997) Effect von Aminfluorid-Zahnpasten auf überemp-findliche Zahnhälse, Acta Med Dent Helv 2:1–5. www.gaba.com/.../Renggli-H-H-1997-Effekt-von-Aminfluorid-Zahnpast. Accessed September 2012

Renton-Harper P, Midda M (1992) NdYAG laser treatment of dentinal hypersensitivity. Br Dent J 172(1):13–6

Ritter AV, de Dias LW, Miguez P, Caplan DJ, Swift EJ Jr (2006) Treating cervical dentin hypersensitivity with fluoride varnish: a randomized clinical study. J Am Dent Assoc 137(7):1013–20

Rosaiah K, Aruna K (2011) Clinical efficacy of amorphous calcium phosphate, G.C. Tooth Mousse and Gluma Desensitizer in treating dentin hypersensitivity. Int J Dent Clin 3(1):1–4

Salvato AR, Clark GE, Gingold J, Curro FA (1992) Clinical effectiveness of a dentifrice containing potassium chloride as a desensitizing agent. Am J Dent 5(6):303–6

Scherman A, Jacobsen PL (1992) Managing dentin hypersensitivity: what treatment to recommend to patients. J Am Dent Assoc 123(4):57–61

Schiff T, Dotson M, Cohen S, de Vizio W, McCool J, Volpe A (1994) Efficacy of a dentifrice containing potassium nitrate, soluble pyrophosphate, PVM/MA copolymer and sodium fluoride on dentine hypersensitivity: a twelve-week clinical study. J Clin Dent 5(Special issue):87–92

Schiff T, Dos Santos M, Laff S, Yoshioka M, Baines E, McCool J, De Vizio W (1998) Efficacy of a dentifrice containing 5% potassium nitrate and 1500 ppm sodium monofluorophosphate in a precipitated calcium carbonate base on dentinal hypersensitivity. J Clin Dent 9:22–25

Schiff T, Zhang YP, De Vizio W, Stewart B, Chaknis P, Petrone ME et al (2000) A randomized clinical trial of the desensitizing efficacy of three dentifrices. Compend Contin Educ Dent Suppl 27:4–10

Schiff T, Delgado E, Zhang YP, DeVizio W, Mateo LR (2009) Clinical evaluation of the efficacy of an in-office desensitizing paste containing 8% arginine and calcium carbonate in providing instant and lasting relief of dentin hypersensitivity. Am J Dent 22(special issue):8A–15A

Schwarz F, Arweiler N, Georg T, Reich E (2002) Desensitizing effects of an Er:YAG laser on hypersensitive dentine. J Clin Periodontol 29(3):211–5

Sharma N, Roy S, Kakar A, Greenspan DC, Scott R (2010) A clinical study comparing oral formulations containing 7.5% calcium sodium phosphosilicate (NovaMin), 5% potassium nitrate, and 0.4% stannous fluoride for the management of dentin hypersensitivity. J Clin Dent 21:88–92

Shetty S, Kohad R, Yeltiwar R (2010) Hydroxyapatite as an in-office agent for tooth hypersensitivity: a clinical and scanning electron microscopic study. J Periodontol 81(12):1781–9

Silverman G (1985) The sensitivity-reducing effect of brushing with a potassium nitrate-sodium monofluorophosphate dentifrice. Compend Contin Educ Dent 6:131–133

Silverman G, Gingold J, Curro FA (1994) Desensitizing effect of a potassium chloride dentifrice. Am J Dent 7:9–12

Silverman G, Berman E, Hanna CB, Salvato A, Fratarcangelo P, Bartizek RD, Bollmer BW, Campbell SL, Lanzalaco AC, Mackay BJ, McClanahan SF, Perlich MA, Shaffer JB (1996) Assessing the efficacy of three dentifrices in the treatment of dentinal hypersensitivity. J Am Dent Assoc 127(2):191–201

Sowinski JA, Battista GW, Pettrone ME, Chaknis P, Zhang YP, DeVizio W et al (2000) A new desensitizing dentifrice: an 8-week clinical investigation. Compend Contin Educ Dent Suppl 27:11–16

Sowinski J, Ayad F, Petrone M, DeVizio W, Volpe A, Ellwood R et al (2001) Comparative investigations of the desensitizing efficacy of a new dentifrice. J Clin Periodontol 28:1032–1036

Starr CB, Mayhew RB, Pierson WP (1989) The efficacy of hypnosis in the treatment of dentin hypersensitivity. Gen Dent 37(1):13–5

Stewardson DA, Crisp RJ, McHugh S, Lendenmann U, Burke FJ (2004) The Effectiveness of Systemp.desensitizer in the treatment of dentine hypersensitivity. Prim Dent Care 11(3):71–6

Swift EJ Jr, May KN Jr, Mitchell S (2001) Clinical evaluation of Prime & Bond 2.1 for treating cervical dentin hypersensitivity. Am J Dent 14(1):13–6

Tantbirojn D, Poolthong S, Leevailoj C, Srisawasdi S, Hodges JS, Randall RC (2006) Clinical evaluation of a resin-modified glass-ionomer liner for cervical dentin hypersensitivity treatment. Am J Dent 19(1):56–60

Tarbet WJ, Silverman G, Stolman JM, Fratarcangelo PA (1980) Clinical evaluation of a new treatment for dentinal hypersensitivity. J Clin Periodontol 51:535–40

Tarbet WJ, Buckner A, Stark MM et al (1981) The pulpal effects of brushing with 5 percent potassium nitrate paste used for desensitization. Oral Surg Oral Med Oral Pathology 51:600–02

Thrash WJ, Jones DL, Dodds WJ (1992) Effect of a fluoride solution on dentinal hypersensitivity. Am J Dent 5(6):299–302

Uchida A, Wakano Y, Fukuyama O, Miki T, Iwayama Y, Okada H (1980) Controlled clinical evaluation of a 10% strontium chloride dentifrice in treatment of dentin hypersensitivity following periodontal surgery. J Periodontol 51:578–81

Umberto R, Claudia R, Gaspare P, Tenore G, Alessandro DV (2012) Treatment of dentine hypersensitivity by diode laser: a clinical study. Int J Dent 2012:Article ID 858950, 8 pages

von Troil B, Needleman I, Sanz M (2002) A systematic review of the prevalence of root sensitivity following periodontal therapy. J Clin Periodontol 29(Suppl 3): 173–7

Walsh T, Worthington HV, Glenny AM, Appelbe P, Marinho VCC, Shi X (2010) Fluoride toothpastes of different concentration for preventing dental caries in children and adolescents. Cochrane Database Syst Rev Issue 1. Art no.:CD007868. doi:10.1002/14651858.CD007868.pub2

Wara-aswapati N, Krongnawakul D, Jiraviboon D, Adulyanon S, Karimbux N, Pitiphat W (2005) The effect of a new toothpaste containing potassium nitrate and triclosan on gingival health, plaque formation and dentine hypersensitivity. J Clin Periodontol 32:53–58

West NX (2007) The dentine hypersensitivity patient – a total management package. Int Dent J 57(Suppl 1):411–419

West NX, Addy M, Jackson RJ, Ridge DB (1997) Dentine hypersensitivity and the placebo response. A comparison of the effect of strontium acetate, potassium nitrate and fluoride toothpastes. J Clin Periodontol 24(4): 209–15

Yates R, West NX, Addy M, Marlow I (1998) The effects of a potassium citrate, cetylpyridinium, sodium fluoride mouthrinse on dentine hypersensitivity, plaque and gingivitis. J Clin Periodontol 25:813–820

Yates R, Ferro R, Newcombe RG, Addy M (2005) A comparison of a reformulated potassium citrate desensitizing toothpaste with the original proprietary product. J Dent 33:19–25

Yengopal V, Mickenautsch S (2009) Caries preventive effect of casein phosphopeptide-amorphous calcium phosphate (CPP-ACP): a meta-analysis. Acta Odontol Scand 67(6):321–32

Yilmaz HG, Kurtulmus-Yilmaz S, Cengiz E, Bayindir H, Aykac Y (2011a) Clinical evaluation of Er, Cr:YSGG and GaAlAs laser therapy for treating dentine hypersensitivity: a randomized controlled clinical trial. J Dent 39(3):249–54

Yilmaz HG, Cengiz E, Kurtulmus-Yilmaz S, Leblebicioglu B (2011b) Effectiveness of Er, Cr:YSGG laser on dentine hypersensitivity: a controlled clinical trial. J Clin Periodontol 38(4):341–6

Zappa U (1994) Self-applied treatments in the management of dentine hypersensitivity. Arch Oral Biol 39(Supplement):107S–112S

Zappa U (1999) The effect of elmex SENSITIVE rinse on hypersensitive teeth. www.gaba.com/download/htm/1211/en/Studie-Zappa-1999.pdf. Accessed September 2012

7 Evaluating Study Designs to Investigate Dentin Hypersensitivity

Sahar Taha and Brian H. Clarkson

Abstract

Studies for investigating dentin hypersensitivity are either epidemiological or testing for the effectiveness of a possible treatment. The latter can be tested in vitro or in vivo. The myriad number of studies evaluating possible treatments for the condition mandates the adoption of rigid criteria for the conduction of such studies in order to validate their results. Literature will be reviewed in this chapter to evaluate the different testing methods for the effectiveness of dentin hypersensitivity treatments.

7.1 Introduction

Studies for investigating dentin hypersensitivity are either epidemiological or testing for the effectiveness of a possible treatment. The latter can be tested in vitro or in vivo. The myriad number of studies evaluating possible treatments for the condition mandates the adoption of rigid criteria for the conduction of such studies in order to validate their results. As mentioned in Chap. 5, the treatment of dentin hypersensitivity is based on its etiology. The obstruction of dentinal tubules after the application of a certain treatment is usually evaluated on dentin sections in vitro. On the other hand, nerve desensitization should be evaluated in vivo using subjective pain scales. Overall, the parameter that needs to be tested dictates the study design.

7.2 Epidemiological Studies

Questionnaires are abundantly used to evaluating the prevalence of dentin hypersensitivity. Results from different studies vary greatly (Table 1.1) and this can be attributed to:

- Lack of a universally agreed on questionnaire for evaluating the condition. All questionnaires should go through an objective process of validation before they can be used on a large scale.
- Sample selection: Many studies evaluated the prevalence of this condition among patients treated at periodontal specialty clinics which overestimated the prevalence values of these studies. Clear inclusion/exclusion criteria should also be adopted in the studies.

S. Taha, DDS, MS, Diplomate (ABOD) (✉)
Department of Conservative Dentistry, Faculty of Dentistry, University of Jordan, 13795, Amman 11942, Jordan
e-mail: shr_taha@yahoo.com, staha@ju.edu.jo

B.H. Clarkson, BChD, LDS, MS, PhD
Department of Cariology, Restorative Sciences and Endodontics, University of Michigan School of Dentistry, 1011, North University, Ann Arbor, MI 48109, USA
e-mail: bricla@umich.edu

S. Taha, B.H. Clarkson (eds.), *Clinician's Guide to the Diagnosis and Management of Tooth Sensitivity*, DOI 10.1007/978-3-642-45164-5_7, © Springer-Verlag Berlin Heidelberg 2014

- Many questionnaires did not correlate the prevalence of this condition with its etiological and predisposing factors, which makes drawing relative conclusions erroneous.

Performing a clinical examination in addition to the questionnaire reduces the shortcomings of the aforementioned study design. Methods used for diagnosing DH clinically are discussed in Chap. 4. In addition, the study of the impact of DH on the quality of life adds more insightful information regarding the effect of this condition and the need for treatment.

7.3 Laboratory Testing

Two main methods have been used for the in vitro evaluation of potential dentin desensitizing agents: scanning electron microscope (SEM) analysis of dentin sections and permeability studies.

Scanning electron microscope images of dentin sections have been evaluated for the obstruction of the dentinal tubules. This method uses a readily available and reproducible test substrate; however, careful attention to the details is mandatory to avoid potential errors. Several previous studies have used dentin discs for the SEM testing (Abed et al. 2011; Thanatvarakorn et al. 2013; Lynch et al. 2012; Earl et al. 2011; Sauro et al. 2006; Pereira et al. 2005; Gillam et al. 1999). Mordan et al. (1997) examined the applicability of the dentin disc as a model for the in vitro testing of DH. They found that dentinal tubules from different dentin discs or even in the same disc have variable morphology. The authors attributed that to two factors: the changes in diameter, orientation, and density of the dentinal tubules throughout the tooth and the relation of the area of the cut to the smear layer morphology. Controls have not always been used in DH studies. However, some studies used control SEM images from the same tooth as the test disc or from a different tooth. Alternatively, many trials covered the control side on the same test disc with barriers like tapes and varnishes. Nevertheless, these methods have not always been successful. Mordan suggested that the dentin disc be halved after etching the sample and preparing it for the treatment. Afterwards, the halves should be mounted as close as possible to each other for SEM analysis. This way, similar areas of dentin can be examined from both the test and control areas in an attempt to overcome the morphological variation. The study also suggested the dentinal tubules in the center of the disc be examined, as they were more circular than dentinal tubules at the periphery (dentin tubules at the peripheries are obliquely cut due to their orientation). Jain et al., in a qualitative study, devised a methodology to overcome tubule variation, whereby a dentin disc was prepared for SEM, imaged, treated, and once again prepared for SEM (Jain et al. 1997). However, the desiccation and gold coating of the disc before treatment and the difficulty in precisely relocating the same area may make this a less realistic model for quantitative studies. The use of an environmental SEM would negate the need to dry and coat the samples, thus the ability to use the same sample as a control and a test is applicable. However, this type of instrument is not readily available and the samples cannot be examined at a later date, because the sections will be altered with the treatments rendered.

The interpretation of the resulting SEM images and drawing relevant conclusions has been challenging. Many hypersensitivity studies (Gillam et al. 1999; Suge et al. 2008; Sauro et al. 2006; Dijkman et al. 1994) relied on subjective evaluation of the images, where the examiners compared the resultant images before and after treatment and ranked the treatments in terms of the "best to worst" coverage of the tubules. No specific criteria were quoted for either what is considered a good coverage, or the degree of dentinal tubule obstruction. This method entails a huge examiner bias and casts doubt on the accuracy of the evaluation. Some attempts have been made to quantify the coverage achieved with the desensitizing agents. Ahmed et al. developed an analysis method for SEM images using automated digital image analysis software (Ahmed et al. 2005). Four micrographs of the control and four corresponding test images were taken at a constant magnification of 1,000X. The images were then analyzed with the Image-Pro Plus software. The gray scale used ranged from 0=black to 255=white, and a level was chosen for the threshold such that only the tubules were highlighted. This threshold could be determined automatically or manually. However, automatic determination was more accurate and

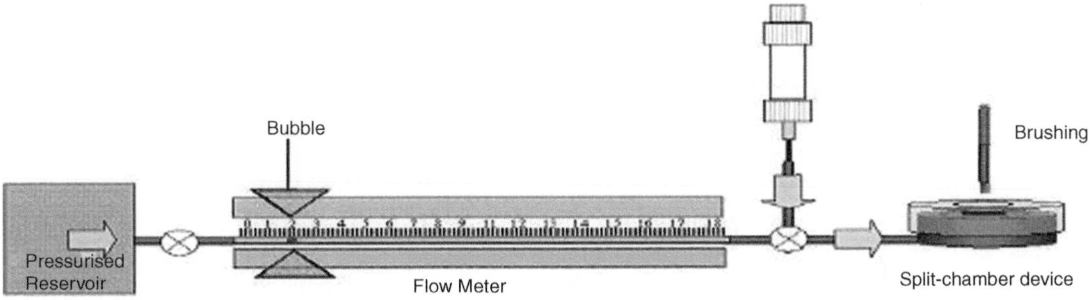

Fig. 7.1 Experimental setup: Dentin discs are placed pulpal side down in a split chamber device. Hydrostatic pressure is applied to the dentin disc via the bottom inlet port by increasing the pressure inside the pressure vessel containing the fluid reservoir

reproducible. Minimum and maximum diameters of the dentinal tubules were calculated using the software. The authors claimed the methodology used in this study was reliable and reproducible with no significant differences within or between the examiners. They emphasized the importance of appropriate statistical analysis as it was shown that neglecting the complexity of clustered data, as often found in studies of this type, could lead to erroneous results and conclusions. It is probable that such measurements were accurate, but this method may be prone to bias and error, as the determination of the areas of interest for conducting the digital analysis is examiner dependent.

Permeability studies of dentin sections have been used extensively to test desensitizing treatments. These studies rely on the ability of the desensitizing treatment applied to the dentin surface to prevent the conductance of fluid through the dentinal tubules of the dentin section. One of the advantages of this method is that the dentin section acts as its own control. After a stabilization period allowing the hydrostatic pressure to increase to 1 psi, the flow rate through the dentin disc is measured (control); the desensitizing treatment is then applied and the conductance is remeasured (experimental). The experimental setup is described below (Fig. 7.1).

The bottom portion of the split chamber device which contains the dentin section is closed except for a single port connected to a fluid reservoir, containing usually Earles' solution, and the top portion of the chamber is open. Hydrostatic pressure is applied to the dentin disc via the bottom inlet port by increasing the pressure inside the pressure vessel to 1 psi. After the stabilization period, the flow rate through both the control and experimental sections is independently measured using a bubble flow meter.

7.4 Clinical Trials

Many clinical trials were conducted to evaluate different treatments for dentin hypersensitivity; however, the methods used and results reported were sometimes contradictory. In addition, the variability of the study methods makes the comparison between different products difficult. It is widely recognized that there is a need to rationalize testing methods and to establish a bench mark for future testing and evaluation of methods for treating dentin hypersensitivity (Holland et al. 1997).

In 1994, a committee was set up comprising academics, clinical specialists, and industrial representatives who had interest in the subject of dentin hypersensitivity and its clinical testing. The committee reported guidelines for conducting clinical trials and set many recommendations for proper testing for DH (Holland et al. 1997). Below is a summary of these recommendations:

- Clinical measurement, data collection, and documentation should be in accordance with FDA and European guidelines for Good Clinical Practice.
- A double-blind, randomized, parallel group design is recommended although the crossover design may be used for the preliminary screening of agents.

- A proper diagnosis of the condition is necessary for subject selection. As DH has many differential diagnoses, it is essential to rule out the various conditions which can be confused with DH (refer to Chap. 4).
- The facial surfaces of permanent incisors, canines, and premolars are the mostly recommended teeth and surfaces for clinical testing.
- Tactile, cold, and evaporative stimuli are the recommended tests for diagnosing DH as these tests are physiologic and controllable.
- At least two hydrodynamic stimuli should be employed starting with the least painful stimulus. It is also very important to leave enough time between applications to minimize the interaction between stimuli.
- Calibration is mandatory for multiple evaluators. Alternatively, each subject should be followed by the same evaluator, or the same stimulus should be applied to all subjects by the same evaluator.
- Controversy exists on the use of controls in the clinical trials. Despite their essentialism in clinical trials, there has not been a consensus on the type of controls to be used. The type and aim of the study should dictate the type of control to be used.
- A run-in/washout period is recommended before the testing starts in order to standardize the subjects and eliminate any already existing effects.
- Eight-week median duration for the clinical trials was reported. However, the duration should vary depending on pilot testing.
- Assessment of the response or treatment results can be stimulus based, which involves measurement of pain threshold, or response-based which involves measuring severity of pain evoked.
- The main objective should be to produce a clinically significant reduction in symptoms rather than a small but statistically significant reduction.
- At least two adequate, well-controlled independent clinical trials should be conducted to demonstrate safety and efficacy of an agent or product before that product receives approval or endorsement by regulatory agencies.

References

Abed AM, Mahdian M, Seifi M, Ziaei SA, Shamsaei M (2011) Comparative assessment of the sealing ability of Nd:YAG laser versus a new desensitizing agent in human dentinal tubules: a pilot study. Odontology 99(1):45–48. doi:10.1007/s10266-010-0136-1

Ahmed TR, Mordan NJ, Gilthorpe MS, Gillam DG (2005) In vitro quantification of changes in human dentine tubule parameters using SEM and digital analysis. J Oral Rehabil 32(8):589–597. doi:10.1111/j.1365-2842.2005.01473.x, JOR1473 [pii]

Dijkman GE, Jongebloed WL, de Vries J, Ogaard B, Arends J (1994) Closing of dentinal tubules by glutaraldehyde treatment, a scanning electron microscopy study. Scand J Dent Res 102(3):144–150

Earl JS, Leary RK, Muller KH, Langford RM, Greenspan DC (2011) Physical and chemical characterization of dentin surface following treatment with NovaMin technology. J Clin Dent 22(3):62–67

Gillam DG, Khan N, Mordan NJ, Barber PM (1999) Scanning electron microscopy (SEM) investigation of selected desensitizing agents in the dentine disc model. Endod Dent Traumatol 15(5):198–204

Holland GR, Narhi MN, Addy M, Gangarosa L, Orchardson R (1997) Guidelines for the design and conduct of clinical trials on dentine hypersensitivity. J Clin Periodontol 24(11):808–813

Jain P, Vargas MA, Denehy GE, Boyer DB (1997) Dentin desensitizing agents: SEM and X-ray microanalysis assessment. Am J Dent 10(1):21–26

Lynch E, Brauer DS, Karpukhina N, Gillam DG, Hill RG (2012) Multi-component bioactive glasses of varying fluoride content for treating dentin hypersensitivity. Dent Mater 28(2):168–178. doi:10.1016/j.dental.2011.11.021, S0109-5641(11)00922-5 [pii]

Mordan NJ, Barber PM, Gillam DG (1997) The dentine disc. A review of its applicability as a model for the in vitro testing of dentine hypersensitivity. J Oral Rehabil 24(2):148–156

Pereira JC, Segala AD, Gillam DG (2005) Effect of desensitizing agents on the hydraulic conductance of human dentin subjected to different surface pre-treatments – an in vitro study. Dent Mater 21(2):129–138. doi:10.1016/j.dental.2004.02.007, S0109564104000417 [pii]

Sauro S, Gandolfi MG, Prati C, Mongiorgi R (2006) Oxalate-containing phytocomplexes as dentine desensitisers: an in vitro study. Arch Oral Biol 51(8):655–664. doi:10.1016/j.archoralbio.2006.02.010, S0003-9969(06)00038-0 [pii]

Suge T, Kawasaki A, Ishikawa K, Matsuo T, Ebisu S (2008) Ammonium hexafluorosilicate elicits calcium phosphate precipitation and shows continuous dentin tubule occlusion. Dent Mater 24(2):192–198. doi:10.1016/j.dental.2007.03.009, S0109-5641(07)00082-6 [pii]

Thanatvarakorn O, Nakashima S, Sadr A, Prasansuttiporn T, Ikeda M, Tagami J (2013) In vitro evaluation of dentinal hydraulic conductance and tubule sealing by a novel calcium-phosphate desensitizer. J Biomed Mater Res B Appl Biomater 101(2):303–309. doi:10.1002/jbm.b.32840

Future Directions for the Treatment of Dentin Hypersensitivity

8

Agata Czajka-Jakubowska and Brian H. Clarkson

Abstract

There are over 30 different treatments for sensitive dentin on the market today which suggests that not one of them gives the immediate and lasting relief from this condition desired by the patient. In this chapter we describe several, emerging, novel experimental technologies that may, in the future, offer such relief. These technologies include: a synthetic "glue" resembling the adhesive that adheres mollusks to rocks in the ocean; a self-etch resin filled with fluorhydroxyapatite (FA) crystrals; and a flexible laminate of Eudragit filled with the FA srystals. Finally the incorporation of dendrimers (artificial proteins) functionalized with anti-inflammatories and anti-microbials to control inflammation beneath sensitive dentin and, overtime, help the pulp repair.

There are over 30 desensitizing products already commercially available for the treatment of dentin hypersensitivity (Amazon.com 2013). The costs of these products vary greatly from \$20–100 per bottle to \$50–260 per desensitizing treatment kit. Several conclusions can be drawn from these two observations. Firstly, dentin hypersensitivity is a problem for a proportion of the general public. Secondly, the public is willing to spend money to alleviate the pain associated with this hypersensitivity. Thirdly, the product ingredients are probably inexpensive, and therefore, the products are profitable. Lastly, and most importantly, there is no "magic bullet" that guarantees immediate and lasting relief from this condition. If there were, there would be only one product or, at the least, a much smaller number than the over 30 now on the market.

The success of any desensitizing therapy, assuming the cause of dentin hypersensitivity, can be explained by the hydrodynamic theory described in Chap. 2, is to prevent the movement of dentinal fluid in patent dentinal tubules. The prevention of this pain can be achieved in two ways by depolarizing the pulpal nerve endings which extend into the dentinal tubules and/or

A. Czajka-Jakubowska (✉)
Department of Maxillofacial Orthopaedics and Orthodontics, Poznan University of Medical Sciences, Poznan, Poland
e-mail: czajak@it.pl

B.H. Clarkson
Department of Cariology, Restorative Sciences and Endodontics, University of Michigan School of Dentistry, Ann Arbor, MI, USA
e-mail: bricla@ju.edu.jo

S. Taha, B.H. Clarkson (eds.), *Clinician's Guide to the Diagnosis and Management of Tooth Sensitivity*, DOI 10.1007/978-3-642-45164-5_8, © Springer-Verlag Berlin Heidelberg 2014 occluding or narrowing the dentinal tubule apertures exposed to the oral environment. Recently, treatments for dentin hypersensitivity appear to be focused on the second therapeutic modality. In order to achieve this, a solution, gel, paste that physically blocks the tubules or causes precipitates to form in the tubules or encourages the formation of peritubular dentin would be an ideal desensitizing therapy. However, these desensitizing agents have to be able to overcome certain constraints if they are to be effective. They have to be non-toxic; able to produce the desired effect in moist conditions; able to withstand positive pressure from the dentinal fluid flow; be substantive, able to withstand eating, drinking, and toothbrushing; and, if possible, be self-applied. Perhaps, the most difficult and most important outcome of a treatment for dentin hypersensitivity is to attain the immediate elimination of the pain associated with this condition with one treatment, and if the one treatment does not give lasting relief, then this should be achieved by multiple treatments.

Recently several new or reengineered products have appeared on the market which include: Sensodyne Repair and Protect with 5–7.5 % NovaMin (a bioglass) and sodium monofluorophosphate (1,450 ppm fluoride); Sensitive Pro-Relief with 8 % arginine, calcium carbonate, and sodium fluoride (1,450 ppm fluoride); ClinPro Tooth Crème with calcium carbonate and calcium phosphate; and a paste with a peptide, MI paste with recaldent. All of these claim incremental reductions in tooth sensitivity overtime but lack the immediate pain relief sought by most patients. There is one study claiming significant, immediate relief and that is using 100 % NovaMin as the desensitizing agent (Narungdej et al. 2010). However this finding needs to be collaborated in further clinical trials.

The arginine and NovaMin technologies are certainly interesting, and the ability of bioglass to produce a calcium phosphate hydroxycarbonate apatite adherent layer, under moist conditions, on dentin surfaces is a novel property. However, even these technologies do not offer the "magic bullet" of immediate and lasting pain relief after one application.

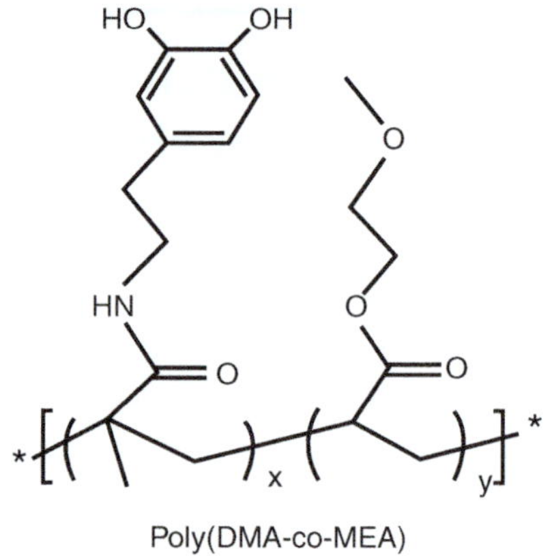

Fig. 8.1 Poly(DMA-co-MEA)

In search of a desensitizing therapy that would offer an immediate and a long-term treatment for dentin hypersensitivity, a self-applied, non-toxic paste that would adhere to wet surfaces would be an ideal carrier for agents that would occlude and then encourage permanent closure of the patent dentinal tubules. Such carriers are synthetic polymers that mimic the "glue" that helps mollusks stick to rocks in the ocean and enables geckos to climb up walls. One such polymer is poly(dopamine methacrylamide-co-methoxyethyl acrylate) [poly(DMA-co-MEA)] (Fig. 8.1). This is a sticky, gelatinous substance that is able to adhere to wet surfaces, an ideal carrier for a dentinal tubule blocking agent. The filler for this polymer needs to be small enough to penetrate into the dentinal tubules which have a diameter of approximately 2u and be bioactive rather than inert. Such bioactivity could be that it produces, when applied to the dentin surface in the oral cavity, a mineralized layer that would help bring about permanent relief of the pain caused by dentin hypersensitivity. In 2006 Chen et al. synthesized fluorhydroxyapatite crystals which resembled enamel crystals in shape, size, and composition. These crystals when produced under ambient conditions were 300–600 nm in length and 50–60 nm in cross section (Fig. 8.2). These crystals were recognized as being ideal as a filler for the poly(DMA-co-MEA) polymer, being of appropriate size and having the possibility to release calcium, phosphate, and fluoride at acid pH.

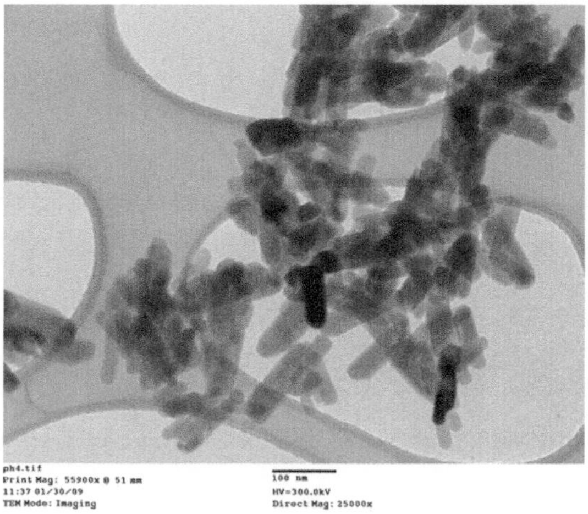

Fig. 8.2 Fluorhydroxyapatite crystals (*FA*). Individual crystals 50–150 nm in length and 20 nm in cross section

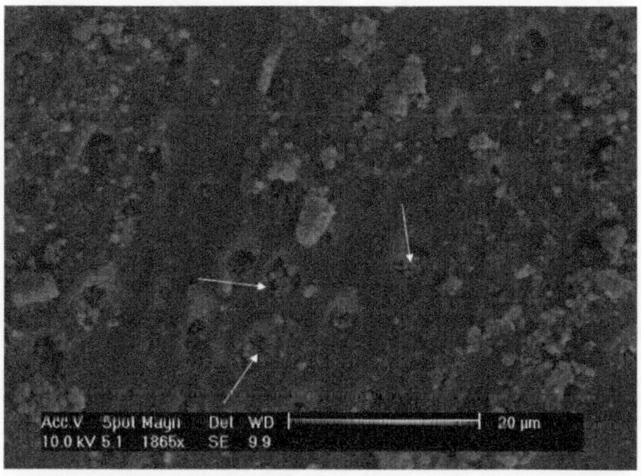

Fig. 8.3 Poly(DMA-co-MEA) + FA crystals obstructing patent tubules. *Arrows* indicate obstruction of dentinal tubule orifice by FA crystals

Thus, over time, in the oral environment, they would have the potential to form a mineralized layer on the dentin surface.

These crystals were incorporated into a poly(DMA-co-MEA) polymer at a fill ratio of 40 % FA (w/v) and the paste applied to wet, EDTA-etched dentin surfaces. The surfaces were then rinsed for 1 min before being viewed in a scanning electron microscope (SEM). The SEM images showed a greater than 80 % obstruction or partial obstruction of the dentinal tubules (Fig. 8.3). This suggests that the paste may produce immediate relief of the symptoms of dentin hypersensitivity after one application. For longer-term relief the paste was tested for ion release under neutral and acid conditions. Calcium, phosphate, and fluoride were released under both of these conditions suggesting that the paste would release the ions under a wide range of intraoral pH. This might then allow for a mineralized layer to form on the surface of the dentin offering permanent, long-term relief of the pain associated with dentin hypersensitivity. A standard XTT assay for toxicity of the poly(DMA-co-MEA) alone and the FA/poly (DMA-co-MEA) paste showed that they were non-toxic. Further work on this novel, experimental desensitizing paste needs to be carried out, especially conductivity tests.

Sealing of the dentin surfaces using a resin has been tried as a cure for dentin hypersensitivity. Unfortunately the drying and etching of the dentin is very uncomfortable for the patient, and long-lasting retention of the resins has been a problem (Duran and Sengun 2004). However, more recently with the advent of the self-etch resins which are more tolerant of the moist conditions in the oral cavity make their use realistic as a carrier for dentinal tubule occluding agents (Ferracane 2011). Thus, we have combined the crystal technology used above with a self-etch resin to produce a dentin desensitizing agent. This paint-on "enamel" has certain advantages over and above the fact that it adheres strongly to dentin surfaces. Both the resin and the FA crystal filler will block the patent dentinal tubules (Fig. 8.4); it can be white or tooth colored to give an esthetic result (Fig. 8.5); and it can be professionally or self-applied depending on the curing mechanism. Perhaps most importantly the self-etch resins are already in clinical use and the FA crystals are similar to enamel crystals, so approval by the Federal Drug Administration should not be a problem. The blockage of the patent tubules by the resin and the FA crystals should offer immediate pain relief with the longer-term relief coming from the release of the ions and the formation of a mineralized surface layer on the dentin which may extend into the tubules. In vitro studies have shown a reduction of 80–85 % of the conductance through dentin sections after drying the dentin surface with a cotton bud and treating the exposed surface once and light curing the resin/FA mixture (Table 8.1). In vivo studies are now planned to test the substantively of the paint-on "enamel" to

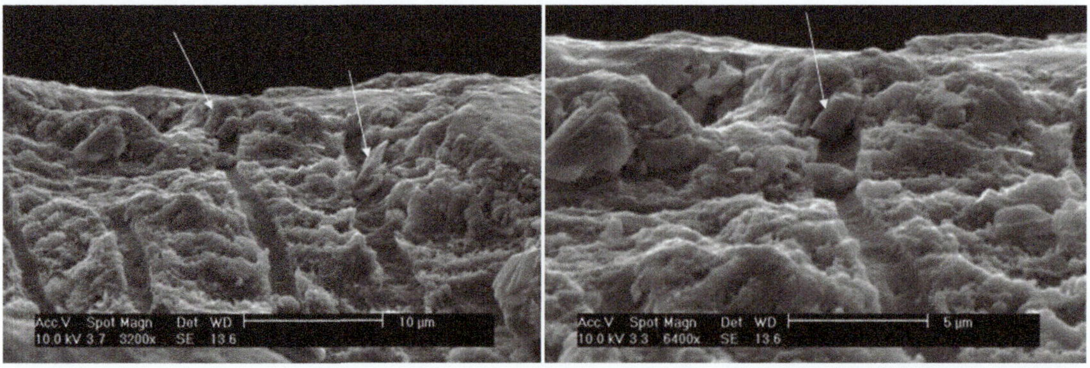

Fig. 8.4 Self-etch resin+FA crystals obstructing the patent dentinal tubules. *Arrows* indicate obstruction of dentinal tubule orifice by FA crystals

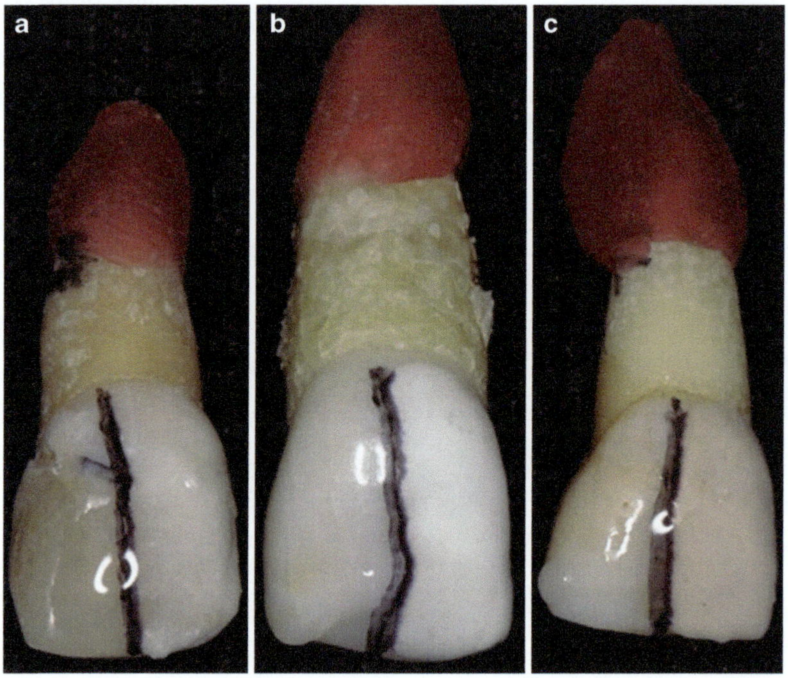

Fig. 8.5 Shows extracted teeth painted with a self-etch resin+FA crystals (paint-on enamel). The paint-on enamel was applied to the right of the black line, and the left on the tooth was remained unpainted. In (**a**) the paint-on enamel was not tinted to match the tooth; in (**b**, **c**) the paint-on enamel was tinted

Table 8.1 Average reduction in hydraulic conductance vs baseline after one application of the self-etch resin+FA (experimental) and H_2O+FA (control) ($N=10$ human dentin discs per treatment)

	One application	
Test product	Mean %	SD
20 % FA in H_2O	23.2	5.3
40 % FA self-adhesive resin	86.1	7.8
20 % FA self-adhesive resin	83.2	9.4

dentin surfaces, and then its ability to give short-term and long-term relief to people suffering from dentin hypersensitivity will be tested.

We have taken the nano-FA crystal technology one step further by creating a flexible nanocrystal laminate using a polymer called Eudragit (Evonik Industries AG) (Fig. 8.6a, b). This substance is used as an enteric coating for tablets, for example, aspirin. The coating prevents the lining of the stomach becoming irritated by the daily consumption of uncoated aspirin tablets. This FA crystal laminate can be of any thickness and be cut using a scalpel or scissors into any shape and size. It is prepared by flowing the Eudragit over a layer of the crystals, allowing the Eudragit to polymerize, and then peeling the FA/Eudragit

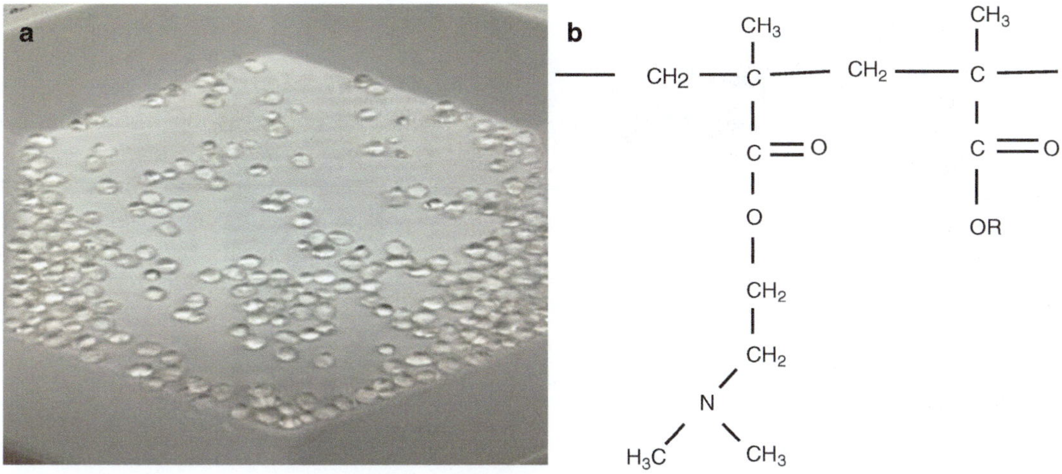

Fig. 8.6 (**a**) Eudragit polymer crystals; (**b**) chemical formula of Eudragit

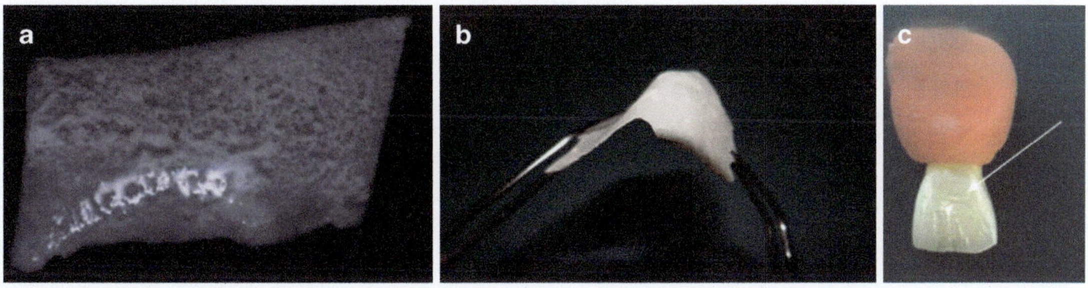

Fig. 8.7 (**a**) Eudragit+FA laminate; (**b**) showing the flexibility of the laminate; (**c**) laminate acid-etched to tooth surface

from the glass or plastic surface. The flexibility of the laminate will allow it to be molded to the curved surfaces of teeth. Once the sensitive area has been identified, the laminate is cut and shaped and bonded to the tooth surface using a self-etch unfilled, light-cured, dental adhesive (Fig. 8.7a–c). The laminate can be tinted to match the tooth, and the self-etch adhesive will bond it to the dentin and adjacent enamel even under moist conditions. The advantage of the laminate over the paint-on "enamel" is that the laminate can be precisely placed, its edges feathered, and the FA crystals will directly contact the tooth surface allowing, over time, the integration of the crystals into the dentin and, perhaps, forming a new enamel surface as the Eudragit dissolves and the adhesive is worn away. Certainly it should provide immediate relief without the pain that may be associated with the drying and etching of sensitive dentin.

Nanoparticles have been a part of medicine for the past 20 years, being used for drug for targeting, in imaging, and as sustained and release on-demand devices. There are several benefits of these particles; they can be as follows: functionalized, positively or negatively charged or neutral, hydrophilic or hydrophobic, nano to micro in size, and release ingredients at specified times and amounts depending on the speed of their degradation.

Dendrimers or artificial proteins are one of the smallest of the nanoparticles 2 nm to 10–15 nm. The size is dependent on the generation number, G1 being the smallest and G2 being larger (Fig. 8.8). These particles are like a tree with a trunk and many branches. It is the branches of the dendrimer that can be functionalized with antimicrobial and or anti-inflammatory agents as suggested by Pashley in Chap. 2. He mentions that dentin tubule-occluding agents should

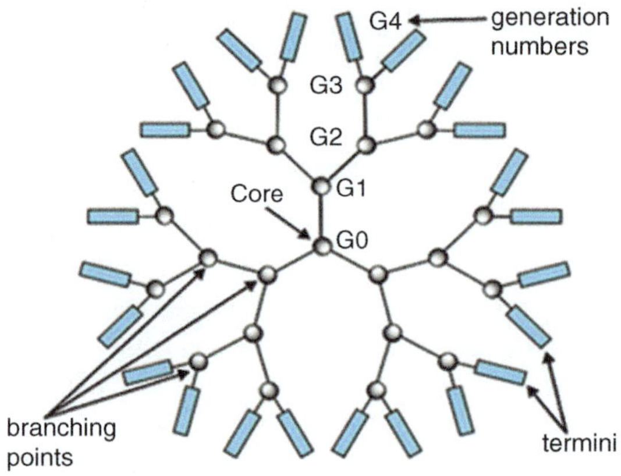

Fig. 8.8 Diagram representation of a generation 4 dendrimer (http://en.wikipedia.org/wiki/File:Graphs.jpg)

include an anti-inflammatory and/or an antimicrobial to control the pulpal inflammation under sensitive dentin to help give immediate and, perhaps, lasting pain relief along with giving time for the pulp to heal. These dendrimers can have any or no charge and be hydrophilic and added to larger particles (100 nm to 1um) in a gel, paste, or liquid and applied to the teeth. The larger particles themselves can be synthesized to contain bioactive ions, for example, calcium, phosphate, and fluoride, that are released as the particle degrades overtime after entering the patent dentinal tubule. Non-toxic, inert particles can also be synthesized which do not degrade but simply block the dentinal tubule. However, even these occluding particles can be made bioactive by coating them with a phosphoprotein or a phosphorylated peptide which is able to attract calcium, and, similar to the degrading particle mentioned earlier, it would catalyze the formation of a calcific barrier (Chang et al. 2006).

References

Tooth desensitizing. Retrieved from http://www.amazon.com. Accessed 1 April 2013

Chang S, Chen H, Liu J, Wood D, Bentley P, Clarkson B (2006) Synthesis of a potentially bioactive hydroxyapatite nucleating molecule. Calcif Tissue Int 78(1):51–61

Chen H, Tang Z, Liu J, Sun K, Chang S-R, Peters T, Czajka-Jakubowska A, Clarkson B (2006) Acellular synthesis of a human-like microstructure. Adv Mater 18(14):1846–1851

Duran I, Sengun A (2004) The long term effect of 5 current desensitising products on cervical dentine sensitivity. J Oral Rehabil 31:351–356

Ferracane J (2011) Resin composite-state of the art. Dent Mater 27(1):29–38

Narungdej T, Sakoolnamarka R, Booroung T (2010) The effectiveness of a calcium phosphosilicate desensitizer in reducing cervical dentin hypersensitivity. J Am Dent Assoc 141:995–999

Index

S. Taha, B.H. Clarkson (eds.), *Clinician's Guide to the Diagnosis and Management of Tooth Sensitivity*, DOI 10.1007/978-3-642-45164-5, © Springer-Verlag Berlin Heidelberg 2014

GPSR Compliance

The European Union's (EU) General Product Safety Regulation (GPSR) is a set of rules that requires consumer products to be safe and our obligations to ensure this.

If you have any concerns about our products, you can contact us on ProductSafety@springernature.com

In case Publisher is established outside the EU, the EU authorized representative is:

Springer Nature Customer Service Center GmbH
Europaplatz 3
69115 Heidelberg, Germany

Batch number: 10683154

Printed by Printforce, the Netherlands